OPIATE ADDICTION

How To Become Drug Free

An unbiased and accurate overview of opiate addiction and its treatment options

To Sonia
I hope you enjoy
my book
Liz
x

Elizabeth Anne Roberts MSc

Orders: Please contact liz.roberts@earconsultancy.co.uk

ISBN: 978-1-5272-6802-9

First published 2020

Disclaimer: Whilst every attempt has been made to ensure the accuracy of the details in this book, information in it should not be relied upon as an alternative to appropriate medical advice. You should consult your doctor or other professional healthcare provider, if you have any specific questions about any medical matter or are suffering from any medical condition, and should not delay seeking medical advice, disregard any medical advice or discontinue any medical intervention because of information contained in this book.

Dedication:

My family

This book is dedicated to my amazing husband David and beautiful daughters, Ali and Katie. Their love and support have meant everything to me and inspired me for more years than I care to remember, even though I may not always have shown it. We have all had to deal with some extremely challenging times, especially recently, but I believe that we are now stronger than ever. No more family secrets!

Susan Elstob

You don't need many friends in life, just the right ones, and anyone that is lucky enough to have a 'Sue' in theirs is fortunate beyond belief. Whilst we share a history of deep sadness, that has not defined our friendship, but merely provided an unbreakable connection few could understand.

PREFACE

'Society's ambivalence towards psychoactive substances is epitomised by the ancient Greek word pharmakon, signifying both medicine and poison – the means both of saving and of taking life. Drugs are taken for the relief of pain, for the treatment of disease, to change mood to soporific euphoria or to hyperactive exuberance, to find or lose identity, to escape, to forget and to explore. The body and sometimes the mind can so crave these sensations that their absence becomes intolerable and drives some users to extremes in order to assuage the desire for more. Others may indulge in occasional or recreational use without ever becoming enslaved. Science has not yet taught us to predict who will become a slave and who a master' (World Drug Report 1997)

Why Me? - I'm not a junkie!

"Why me? Why has my life been blighted by addiction while my friends and family appear to be immune?"

Hello and thank you for picking up a copy of this guide. My name is Elizabeth Roberts, and in this book, I aim to walk you through the causes of opiate addiction and provide you with an unbiased view of the treatment options which may be available. Whilst our bookstores are littered with dozens of 'self-help manuals' or true-life stories of someone's battle with and victory over addiction, what this book aims to deliver is different.

We all frequently see headline grabbing news about the so called 'opioid epidemic' sweeping the United States, especially when it claims the life of yet another high-profile celebrity. Here in the UK, there are increasing warnings that the threat is now taking a foot hold on our shores, and a steady stream of our own home-grown celebrities are coming forward to publicly share their own stories or recommend one technique or treatment over another. But what about the ordinary man or woman on the street, who is not blessed with the financial resources of the rich and famous? Where does he or she go, to not only find support but to find reliable, credible and accurate information on the causes and management of addiction. Despite the freedom the world wide web brings to millions of people around the world, finding accurate and validated information about recovery from opiate addiction that is produced in a format that is easy to digest is surprisingly difficult to find. The maxim 'a little knowledge is a dangerous thing' is very true, especially when that knowledge is often founded upon fake or inaccurate information or influenced by an individual's own preferences or experiences, no matter how well intentioned.

As you work through the chapters in this book, you will be introduced to what is often referred to as 'The Perfect Storm'. In other words, a combination of factors which, when they come together, create that mix of chemical, emotional and social ingredients which are almost always present in addiction. I am fortunate enough to be able to draw upon my own extensive professional, academic and personal experiences, in order to write about such an emotive subject. To gain your trust and respect as an author, I feel that I need to provide you with a little background about what brought me to this point. But as my reader, if you are not interested in this, you are quite at liberty to skip though this part and delve into the meatier aspects of this book instead.

Why I wrote this book

It is important to state at this point that the main aims behind writing this book are simple. The purpose of this book is to explore opioid addiction. I wish to supply accurate and reliable information to people who are not only struggling to get to grips with addiction but are also struggling to find information that is both digestible and will stand up to academic scrutiny. I am driven by the frustration that much of the information available to the people who need it is either incomplete or just plain wrong. I will be sticking with what I know and exploring the causes of addiction and explaining the pros and cons of some of the most widely used medical treatments that are frequently prescribed to manage opioid addiction. I will leave the intricacies of the so-called but essential 'talking therapies' to people far better qualified than I am. This book aims to equip you with sufficient knowledge to help you to make informed choices about why, or why not, certain treatment options may be appropriate.

Professional: I have enjoyed a career working in the addictions and mental health field spanning over 30 years. Through my career in the pharmaceutical industry I have had the privilege of working alongside many eminent clinicians and academics who have shared my passion for this challenging yet rewarding arena. However, this experience was frequently eclipsed by the honour of meeting and getting to know a vast array of people from all walks of life who had (and in some cases are still) battling with addiction. The life journeys of these incredible people have inspired me and proved to me that there is always hope!

Academic: As a young schoolgirl I was never motivated to go to university to get a degree. To the despair of my parents and teachers, at the age of 13, I set my sights firmly on a career in the police force. I pursued this end vigorously until my police career ended abruptly 8 years later, as a result of a serious road traffic accident whilst on duty. Following this disaster, which could have easily ended my life, I was fortunate enough to begin a new career in the pharmaceutical industry and was delighted to find that, like the police force, this career path also provided me with a company car and an opportunity for people to be rude to me! However, my professional experiences finally provided me with sufficient inspiration to take on and complete a Masters in "Drugs and Alcohol: Policies and Interventions" at the Imperial College of Science, Technology and Medicine, London.

Personal: So, with both the 'professional' and 'academic' boxes well and truly ticked, and with a passion for this subject which stems from my own personal experiences both as a child and as an adult, I feel driven to help provide what people need to know. My life has been an emotional roller coaster, with childhood trauma, post-traumatic stress disorder, anxiety disorders and depression being background noise throughout.

Whilst writing this book has forced me to delve into areas of my life I have attempted to close off, I do not write this as a cathartic 'self-help' manual. Although unbelievably, I have avoided the total devastation caused by drug addiction, I have still at times hurtled towards the Black Hole but have miraculously escaped its all-consuming presence by the skin of my teeth and the love of those close to me. No, I am merely driven by the frustration that so much of the information available is either incomplete or just plain wrong.

Managing expectations- there is no quick fix!

As you will come to understand, addiction is a multi-faceted condition requiring a wide variety of approaches and interventions. The take home message is that there is no quick fix. We need to know enough to be able to make informed choices about why certain interventions or treatment options may or may not suit us. A helpful analogy is learning to drive. You will know that there is no substitute for engaging qualified, patient and experienced instructors. Alongside this you will need the support of family and friends as well as plenty of practice. You will also need to develop resilience in order to turn mistakes that you make into opportunities to learn because, after all, many people do not pass their driving test on the first attempt. Bringing all of these factors together is the Highway Code which is derived from experience and which helps you to understand and apply the rules of the road. I hope that you will come to consider this book as an equally useful manual.

It is important to always bear in mind that learning to drive comes a lot easier for some than for others. No two experiences are the same, but the key thing to remember is that if you keep going, nearly everyone passes their test at some point and goes on to become a safe and competent driver. The same is true of addiction.

The 'Legal Stuff'

We will cover a lot of ground together in *Opiate Addiction: How To Become Drug Free,* and I have done my best to make your experience as a reader as engaging as possible. One of the main aims I have in writing this book, is to ensure that the content is as robust as possible. At times however, I found that the more legal and technical aspects hampered the flow of the story I wanted to tell. To overcome this dilemma, I added a new chapter at the end of the book entitled 'Legal Stuff', in which I have gathered together relevant legal information, together with links to key reference documents. Please feel free to treat this as a reference chapter that you can dip in and out of as required.

Recommendations, Resources and Support

I have also included a list of organisations and websites, together with a couple of recommendations for additional reading at the end of the **'Legal Stuff',** which provide you with a wide range of information beyond opioid addiction itself.

Contents

CHAPTER 1

Addiction- What Makes People Succumb?

'The desire to experience some altered state of consciousness seems to be an intrinsic part of the human condition...we are surrounded by drugs... the cup of coffee and tea, the glass of beer, wine or whisky, the cigarettes, the snorts of cocaine, the joints, the tablets of acid, the fixes of heroin and the ubiquitous tranquillisers and sleeping pills. Drug taking still remains one of the easiest and most immediate ways of altering psychological states; for some people, the ease and immediacy with which drugs achieve these effects prove particularly seductive. So long as there are drug takers there will be drug casualties but the quest to eliminate drug taking has proved to be the search for a chimera. Drug taking is here to stay and one way or another we must all learn to live with drugs.' (Gossop 1993)

Why do people use drugs?

Human beings have taken substances for pleasure or for the relief of distress for millennia. Whilst intoxication may pre-date farming, the use of plants for healing purposes goes back even further and forms the origin of much of our modern medicine. In fact, many of our widely used, conventional drugs originate from plant sources such as aspirin (derived from willow bark), digoxin (derived from the foxglove) and of course morphine (derived from the opium poppy).

In these modern times, life expectancy is generally increasing year on year, and in the western world at least, most people get to adulthood in reasonable physical health and enjoy a relatively good standard of living. Unfortunately, improvements in life expectancy have stalled in the United Kingdom over the past decade, and for certain groups of the population, actually gone into reverse. There is a widening gap in life expectancy between the richest and poorest. Those who are fortunate enough to have their basic needs met have more time and resources to spend pursuing pleasurable activities-including consuming drugs. However, on the other side of this coin, there are many people who may or may not have all their basic needs met but who, because of personal circumstances, look to drugs to manage their physical and, most importantly, their emotional needs. We will come to see that the reasons *why* a person uses drugs plays a significant role in addiction.

Today there is an increasing range of mood-enhancing drugs that we use which affect the brain - some are legal, such as caffeine, nicotine and alcohol and others are not, such as cannabis (in many countries), cocaine, heroin, and ecstasy. Some are legal when prescribed but used in ways they were not intended for. This may be referred to as 'unauthorised use'. Unauthorised use of a drug may occur even when it is a medicine that has been prescribed by a doctor or bought 'over-the-counter' by a patient. In these situations, unauthorised use may occur if a medication is prescribed for a patient but is subsequently used by that patient at a different dose, in a different way, or for a different purpose than prescribed; for example, using steroids to enhance performance. Unauthorised use also occurs when a medicine is used by someone other than the intended user.

Aside from performance-enhancing steroids, other medications that are often associated with unauthorised use include the benzodiazepines, which includes diazepam (commonly known by its brand name Valium), and temazepam, which are generally used to treat anxiety and sleep disorders. The so-called Z-drugs (Zopiclone and Zolpidem) are commonly used hypnotics (sleep medicines) and can also cause dependence if used in an unauthorised manner.

However, the most widely misused drugs are the opioids, such as morphine, codeine-based pain relief medications, such as co-codomol, or other opioids including tramadol, buprenorphine, fentanyl and oxycodone. So, in short, drug misuse does not only involve illicit or 'street drugs' such as heroin or cocaine - It can also involve legally prescribed or purchased medicines. The fact that our pharmacy shelves are stocked with licensed and regulated drugs does not mean that they are free from the well-publicised harm associated with 'street drugs'. Because of their high misuse potential, prescriptions for these medications can have a 'street value'. In other words, people intending to use them in an unauthorised way are willing to pay the intended patient for their medication with money, goods or services. It is also not uncommon for the patient to be bullied, assaulted or worse, in order for someone to obtain their medication. These threats to personal safety can often extend to the patient's friends and family too.

What is addiction?

There are many theories and arguments around the causes of addiction. Is it a 'lifestyle choice', is it a disease? Is it genetic? Is it learned behaviour? Have the brain systems been hijacked? Addiction is certainly no respecter of gender, age, wealth, background or culture. Drugs that cause dependence affect parts of the brain involved in decision making, reward, motivation and free will. This can result in impaired judgement and the continued repetitive use of the drug. So, when someone first uses drugs, they are generally able to control their use but for some, continued or prolonged use results in a state of compulsive behaviour which is difficult, but not impossible, to change.

What's in a word?

It is worth spending a few moments exploring the terminology and definitions that exist around addiction. It is extremely difficult to pin down a pure definition, as the term 'addiction' is often used interchangeably with the term 'dependence', and for the person living with the issue, it matters not whether they are considered to be 'addicted to' or 'dependent upon' a particular drug or activity. Historically, the term 'addict' is used as a negative label which places blame on the individual and has served to stigmatise and demonise whole sections of society. Fortunately, many cultures are moving away from this judgmental and damaging approach that labels someone as bad or mad. Today, greater empathy and understanding has led to a subtle shift in language away from the term addict. Instead, phrases such as 'someone who is dependent upon...' or 'someone who is living with addiction' are widely use. There is also a shift away from negative terms such as 'abuse' in favour of the word 'misuse', for example, an individual may be described as 'suffering from a substance misuse disorder'. The softening of the language should not detract from the suffering of the individual or remove their ultimate responsibility in managing their dependence. However, it does attempt to deflect blame away from that person and that is surely a positive thing.

In addition to the humanising of addiction, scientific research has extended a long-overdue hand to people living with addiction, and opened up more treatment options and, whilst no treatment is without side-effects, these interventions and medications have *helped* millions of people journey along the road to recovery.

There are a number of definitions of addictions (commonly referred to as the 'dependence syndrome') which have been published. For example, the *International Classification of Disease (ICD-10)* defines it as:

'A cluster of physiological, behavioural, and cognitive phenomena in which the use of a substance or a class of substances takes on a much higher priority for a given individual than other behaviours that once had greater value. A central descriptive characteristic of the dependence syndrome is the desire (often strong, sometimes overpowering) to take psychoactive drugs (which may or may not have been medically prescribed), alcohol, or tobacco. There may be evidence that return to substance use after a period of abstinence leads to a more rapid reappearance of other features of the syndrome than occurs with nondependent individuals.'

The *National Institute of Drug Abuse (NIDA)* is an American-based research organisation. It defines addiction as:

'A chronic, relapsing disorder characterized by compulsive drug seeking, continued use despite harmful consequences, and long-lasting changes in the brain. It is considered both a complex brain disorder and a mental illness.'

However, neither of these definitions really hit the mark. Neither of them takes into account addictive behaviours, such as gambling, sex, shopping, computer games, use of smart phones etc. but there is no doubt that these activities also fit the criteria and can cause equal devastation to lives. The NIDA definition limits addiction to that of a brain disorder but, as you will see, addiction is so much more than that.

The *Merriam-Webster dictionary* provides a much more useful definition of addiction which not only takes in to account the importance of psychological and social factors, but also includes addictive behaviours:

'Addiction is a compulsive, chronic, physiological or psychological need for a habit-forming substance, behavior, or activity having harmful physical, psychological, or social effects and typically causing well-defined symptoms (such as anxiety, irritability, tremors, or nausea) upon withdrawal or abstinence.'

The Reward Pathway

As human beings, we naturally engage in activities which are vital for our survival as an individual and as a species. These activities are essential to life and include eating, drinking, sex and nurturing. These actions are pleasurable and that is why we repeat them. In effect we receive a kind of 'reward' from the part of the brain involved in motivation and pleasure which is known as the 'reward pathway'. When we engage in certain pleasurable activities, this pathway releases a feel-good chemical called *dopamine* into the brain which *reinforces* how pleasurable the activity was and encourages us to do it again. This is known as '*positive reinforcement*'.

As we have seen, there are rewarding behaviours and activities which are entirely natural, but there are also artificial ones, including using drugs. Some types of drugs directly act on the 'reward pathway', effectively 'hijacking' it to such an extent that, for some people, taking the drug becomes more important than anything else in their life. This *loss of control* or *compulsion* to use, even when faced with negative consequences (even extreme ones), is a key component in both identifying and treating addiction.

'Neuroadaptation'

Neuroadaptation is the term used to describe the brain changes that occur following repeated use of an addictive drug or behavior. Neuroadaptation occurs when the pleasure pathways are repeatedly stimulated by a specific drug or behavior, and in doing so are 'taken over' or 'hijacked'. This leads to the drug or behavior having undue influence over the person, and leads to craving, tolerance, dependence and withdrawal symptoms. Although some effects of neuroadaptation go away when you become abstinent, there are, in people who have been addicted, also long-lasting effects that may not go away. This includes 'residual' brain changes and conditioned responses which can be reactivated following a lapse or relapse.

The Perfect Storm of Addiction

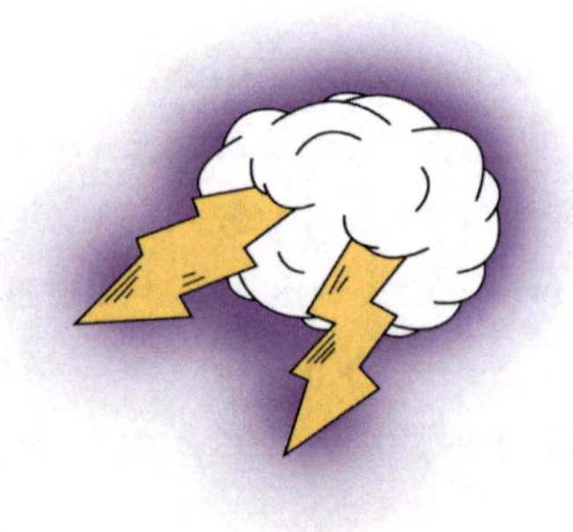

We have just seen that drugs that can cause addiction affect parts of our brain involved in motivation, decision making, reward and pleasure, but that does not explain what makes some people rather than others succumb. In the case of opioids for example, the majority of people just take them for relief from pain and are able to stop when the pain has been managed. Others, on the other hand, will use a variety of means, some legal but many not, to obtain these drugs regardless of the physical, psychological, legal or financial consequences. Scientists now understand more about what happens in the brains of people dependent upon drugs and it is very clear that true addiction is a complex mix of biological, psychological and environmental factors. Dr Norman Earl Zinberg was an American psychiatrist and psychoanalyst who carried out extensive research in the recreational use of heroin. His book, entitled 'Drug, Set, and Setting: The Basis for Controlled Intoxicant Use', which was published in the 1980s, demonstrated that someone's reaction to a drug was far more complex than the drug itself, and could change according to their mindset and social setting. In other words, whether a person becomes addicted will largely depend upon the following 3 factors-

a. The **DRUG** – The drug itself and its effect on the individual, including the type, quantity and manner in which the drug is taken

b. The **SET** – The physical and emotional health, including the mindset and personality of the individual

c. The **SETTING** – The emotional, physical, social and cultural environment in which the drug is being used

So, let's expand a little on the Drug, Set and Setting theory.

a) **The Drug Itself**

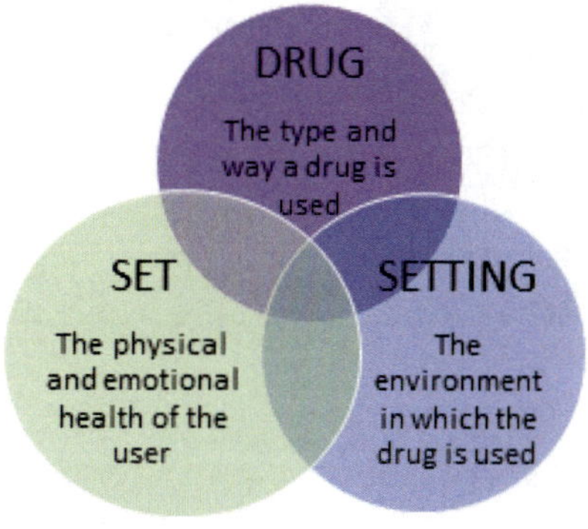

It goes without saying that to become dependent upon, or addicted to drugs, there must be some type of substance that is consumed. Different types of drugs have different effects, and a drug's effect on the reward pathway will play a key part in how addictive it is. To help simplify this, let us put some of the most commonly used drugs into 3 different categories. It is important to note at this point that we are not just referring to illicit or illegal drugs but also drugs with a medicinal use which are either prescribed or purchased over-the-counter.

	'Depressant' Drugs	'Stimulant' Drugs	'Hallucinogenic' Drugs
Effect	Slow down the messages between the brain and the body, which can affect concentration and coordination, as well as cause drowsiness. They do not necessarily make you feel emotionally depressed.	Can cause increased alertness, awareness, wakefulness, endurance, and motivation. Unlike 'depressants', they can increase your heart rate and blood pressure. In high doses, stimulants can cause hallucinations.	Can alter your perception of the world, distort your experience of things, and give you visual, auditory or other sensory hallucinations. May also produce rapid, intense emotional swings.
Examples	Alcohol, benzodiazepines, cannabis, opioids, poppers (inhaled alkyl nitrites)	Amphetamine, cocaine, ecstasy, nicotine	High dose cannabis, L.S.D (Lysergic Acid Diethylamide), ketamine, PCP (phencyclidine)

How the drug is taken

In addition to the drug's effect, the quantity and manner in which it is taken can also have a massive impact on how addictive a drug is and also how harmful it can be. To demonstrate this, I have listed the most widely used routes of administration ranging from the fastest to the slowest. We will cover this in more detail in chapter 3 but in terms of opioid dependence, the faster the route to the brain, the better the high, and the greater the risk of causing dependence.

Methods of drug administration in order of fastest to slowest response

Injecting

There are various ways of injecting a drug into the body and opioids are not only injected in the context of misuse (e.g. injecting 'street drugs'), but also in the management of substance misuse as part of a planned treatment programme (we will look at this more closely in chapter 6), and as part of pain management. There are 3 ways that a drug is injected:

I. Intravenous (IV)

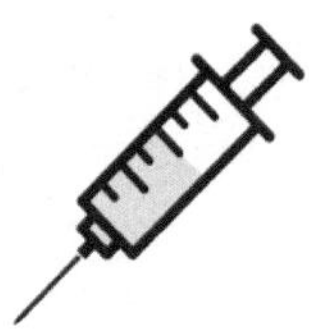

This means that the drug is injected directly into a vein, where it enters the bloodstream and reaches the brain very quickly. This is the quickest route of administration, as the drug's effect is experienced in less than one minute. However, it also carries a high risk of accidental overdose, as well as a high risk of contracting bacterial and viral infections as a result of sharing needles, syringes and other injecting paraphernalia. The term often used for injecting 'street' drugs is 'shooting up', and opioids, such as heroin, are often administered this way.

II. Intramuscular (IM)

Intramuscular injections are delivered into the muscle. The drug effect is not quite as fast as with the intravenous route but may be useful when administering drugs which are irritating to veins, or because a suitable vein cannot be located quickly or at all. It has been demonstrated that in certain emergency situations, the benefits of a quicker onset of drug effect achieved with IV administration is outweighed by the ease and shorter time it takes to administer the IM injection.

III. Subcutaneous (SC)

Subcutaneous injections are administered into the fat layer located underneath the skin and are absorbed slower than intramuscular injections. This is because muscle tissue has a greater blood supply than the tissue just under the skin. Muscle tissue can also hold a larger volume of medication than subcutaneous tissue. SC injecting is commonly called 'skin popping' by drug users, and frequently causes painful lumps ('sterile abscesses') or infected abscesses.

Inhaling/smoking

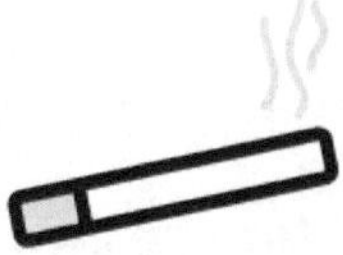

Inhaling substances causes an effect almost as quickly as injecting them because the gaseous vapour passes easily and quickly through the lining of the lungs and into the bloodstream. Inhaling heroin is also known as Chasing the Dragon; heroin is heated, and the fumes are inhaled. This route of administration creates an intense subjective 'high', more intense than sniffing or snorting. It is considered to be an easier and safer method than injecting, both in terms of accidental overdose as the dose can be titrated by the individual, and also in terms of infection risk as there is no sharing of injecting equipment. However, smoking heroin can also be extremely dangerous and can lead to serious respiratory problems, including pneumonia.

Snorting/sniffing

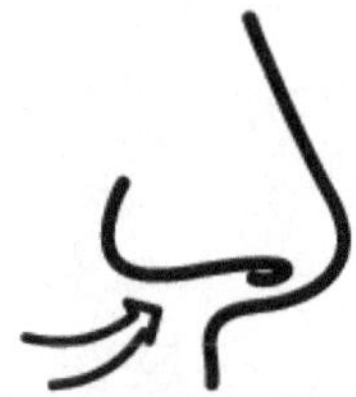

Snorting or sniffing a powdered drug is also an extremely quick route of administration as the effect can be achieved in a couple of minutes. This is because the drug is absorbed quickly through the mucous membranes inside the nose and then into the bloodstream. In addition to heroin, substances which are also commonly snorted include cocaine or amphetamine (speed). Snorting heroin is often the preferred route for individuals who are new to using the drug. The 'high' is not as intense and takes slightly longer than either injecting or inhaling, and there is no injecting equipment or drug using paraphernalia required. However, people often progress to smoking or injecting as their tolerance to the drug increases. We will look more closely at this later on.

Sublingual or Buccal

Sublingual and buccal administration are two different ways of giving medication by mouth. Sublingual administration involves placing a drug under your tongue to dissolve, and buccal administration involves placing the drug between your gums and cheek. The drug is then absorbed quickly into your bloodstream through the tissue there. However, eating, drinking, or smoking can affect how the drug is absorbed and how well it works. The sublingual route of administration of opioid analgesics has been a mainstay in the pain management for patients who are unable to swallow. It is also useful for administering medications when nausea or vomiting is present, or for administering medicines which cannot be swallowed because their effects are either reduced by going via the gut or are broken down by the liver to the extent that they do not work adequately (known as 'first pass hepatic metabolism'). Both sublingual and buccal drugs come in tablets, films, or sprays which are rapidly absorbed. This can also be helpful in settings where there are concerns about the unauthorised use of medication as it makes diverting the medication for use by someone else extremely difficult. The most widely used sublingual opioid is buprenorphine, which is frequently used in the management of both pain and substance misuse disorders.

Oral

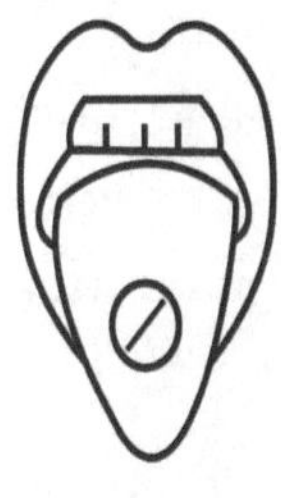

Swallowing a drug is a relatively slow route of administration. After the drug is swallowed, it is dissolved in the stomach and is then absorbed into the bloodstream from the linings of the stomach and the small intestine. Liquid medicines generally produce drug effects in five to ten minutes, but drugs in tablet form can take from half an hour or less, to over an hour for the onset of the drug effect. The time it takes for a drug to be absorbed can also be increased if they are crushed or taken with hot liquids, or reduced if the stomach contains food, which will need to be digested. Some oral formulations are also specifically designed to dissolve in a controlled manner so that they have a smoother onset of effect and last longer – known as modified release formulations. These tablets should not be chewed or crushed but swallowed whole.

Transdermal Patches

Transdermal patches which contain opioids such as buprenorphine are widely used for pain management. The transdermal patch is placed onto the skin and can take several days before the effects are felt, but the effects may then last for as long as a week. Because the build-up of effect is gradual, the reduction in effect will also be gradual, meaning that any opioid withdrawal effects (see chapter 5) should be minimal, if any. The patches may cause skin irritation and, most importantly, should not be exposed to external heating sources, such as radiators, heat lamps or saunas, as the heat will increase the absorption of the drug into the blood stream. This may result in enhanced effects, including an increased risk of side-effects, as well as overdose.

Rectal

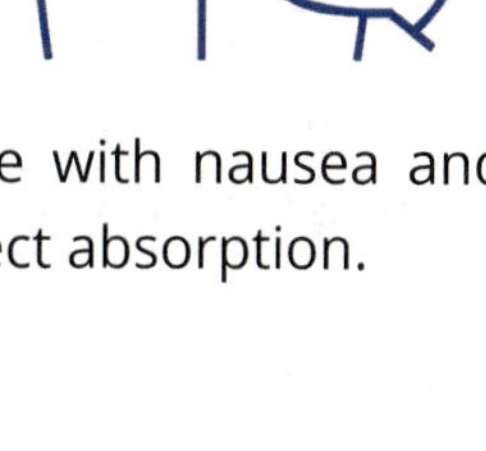

Rectal use of a drug involves the insertion of the drug into the rectum, where it can dissolve slowly and be absorbed into the bloodstream via the linings of the rectum. Rectal administration is rarely used recreationally. It is, however, likely to be performed in a medical setting for patients who cannot swallow, who have trouble with nausea and vomiting or have other conditions which may affect absorption.

b) The Set – Your health and mindset

In addition to the type, quantity and manner in which a drug is taken, your own unique characteristics, including your physical make up, will influence the effect that the drug will have. Factors affecting your response to the drug include your mental, emotional and physical health. Your cultural identity, your sense of belonging and your expectations and motivations for using the drug will also be important. These factors are especially true for people who succumb to opioid addiction as we will see later.

c) The Setting – Your physical and emotional environment

Where and with whom you take the drug will also play a part in your drug-taking experience. This will also include your cultural and social environment.

Your emotional, physical, cultural and social environments do not, of course, stand still. Instead, they change over time. Likewise, your emotional needs and priorities will change as you get older. There has been research that shows that the main factors that lead to a person's recovery is that they became sick and tired of being sick and tired. In effect, they grew tired of the impact that their drug use was having on their quality of life. Changes in spiritual or religious beliefs also played a key role in recovery.

Whilst a theoretical awareness is always useful, it is often more helpful to be able to apply theory to practice. So, to paint a clearer picture, imagine the following 3 scenarios. If you are someone who drinks alcohol, visualise your favorite beverage - perhaps a can or glass of beer, cider or wine. Now, imagine drinking that can or glass at home on a Wednesday evening, watching the news on TV before heading off to bed early as you have work in the morning.

Next, imagine that instead of watching TV you are drinking that can or glass with your friends whilst preparing for a night out.

Finally, imagine drinking that same drink at a wake following the funeral of a loved-one. In all 3 situations, the 'drug' i.e. the can or glass of alcohol, is the same. However, your mind-set in all 3 is different i.e. relaxing, excited or sad. Likewise the setting or environment is different. The likelihood is that the anticipated and actual effect of that drink will therefore be different in all 3 settings. You can also add in additional factors. For example, change that wine or beer to prosecco or champagne, with its association to celebratory occasions and imagine consuming it whilst out with friends, with a meal on a tray in front of the television or at a wake in the presence of strangers from different religious or cultural backgrounds. All of these factors will impact the effect of that same amount of alcohol.

I hope that this chapter has given you a better insight into how complex addiction is. It is not as simple as just taking a particular drug. Various anti-drug media campaigns were shown to be ineffective, as they simply gave an inaccurate message. Slogans like 'one hit and you're hooked' were designed to scare young people and deter them from experimenting. The truth, however, is that 'one hit and your hooked' simply isn't true, as many young people found out for themselves. The result of such failed campaigns not only discredited the authors but exposed some vulnerable young people to the risk of addiction by lulling them into a false sense of security.

Let us now start to look at the role opioids play in creating that perfect storm.

CHAPTER 2
All About Opioids

What are opioids?

In this chapter we will look at opioids, what they are and what they are used for. You may not have come across the term opioid before, so to begin with, let us clear up any confusion:

Opiates	Opioids
Opiates are naturally occurring substances which are extracted from the opium poppy (*Papaver somniferum*) and include morphine, codeine and thebane.	Opioids generally refer to something that mimics the effect of natural opiates but are ***synthetic*** or ***semi-synthetic*** i.e. they have been adapted by humans, and include heroin, methadone and buprenorphine.

Whilst there are people who insist on using the different terms as specified above, most people use the term OPIOID to cover ALL of these compounds. It is easiest to think of opioid as a family name covering all of these compounds, whether natural or synthetic, so from now on, we will use the catch-all term, 'opioid' throughout the book.

I have produced a couple of tables which lists the most commonly used opioids, both legal and illicit. It is worth noting that most medications, including opioids, have 2 names. The first name is known as the 'generic' or 'drug' name, and this will be the name it was given while it was initially being developed by a pharmaceutical company. When a drug receives a licence which permits it to be given to patients (by prescription or for purchase over-the-counter), the pharmaceutical company will give it a 'brand name' which they will use to market the drug. They do this in an attempt to protect their market share. Once the drug's patent has expired, other manufacturers are permitted to copy the drug and 'cash in' on that particular market. Interestingly, a patent lasts for 20 years from the date it is registered with the patent office NOT from the date the licence is granted for use by patients. Getting a drug 'to market' is a complex, costly and time-consuming process and the majority of drugs that are patented are never licensed. Those that do become licensed may only have a few years left before their patent expires because of the rigorous processes that must be completed to ensure that the drug is both safe and effective. This helps to explain why new drugs are often more expensive than older ones, as the manufacturers need to not only recoup their research and development costs for that particular medication, but also for those that failed to reach the market. It also explains why some medications have the same generic name but have a different brand name as you can see from the following tables:

Natural opiates	Some 'Brand' names[1]
Codeine[1]	Co-codamol, Codipar, Kapake, Migraleve, Neurofen Plus, Panadol Ultra, Solpadeine, Solpadol, Syndol, Tylex, Utramol, Zapain
Heroin (diamorphine)	N/A
Morphine	Cyclimorph, J Collis Browne's, Kaolin and Morphine, Morphgesic, MST Continus, MXL, Oramorph, Sevredol, Zomorph
Thebane	None – not marketed

Semi Synthetic & Synthetic	Some 'Brand' names[1]
Buprenorphine	Buvidal, Espranor, Prefebin, Subutex, Suboxone[3]
Di-hydrocodeine	DF118, Paramol[1], DHC Continus
Fentanyl[1]	Duragesic
Heroin (diamorphine)	Ayendi (nasal spray)
Hydrocodone[2]	Lortab
Hydromorphone[2]	Dilaudud, Pallodone
Methadone	Physeptone, Methadose
Oxycodone[2]	IxylR, Norco, Oxycontin
Oxymorphone[2]	Opana, Opana ER (USA)
Tramadol	Tilodol, Maxitram

1. Often combined with other analgesics which increase the risk of toxicity and physical health issues if misused
2. Widely misused in the USA
3. Suboxone® also contains another active ingredient naloxone

What are opioids used for?

The main use for opioids is for the relief of certain types of pain, as they mimic the natural 'feel-good' chemical in our brain called **endorphin.** Millions of people worldwide have benefited from their analgesic properties for millennia.

Opioids can also produce euphoria or pleasurable feelings but can also cause some less desirable side-effects, including **dependence** and ultimately, death.

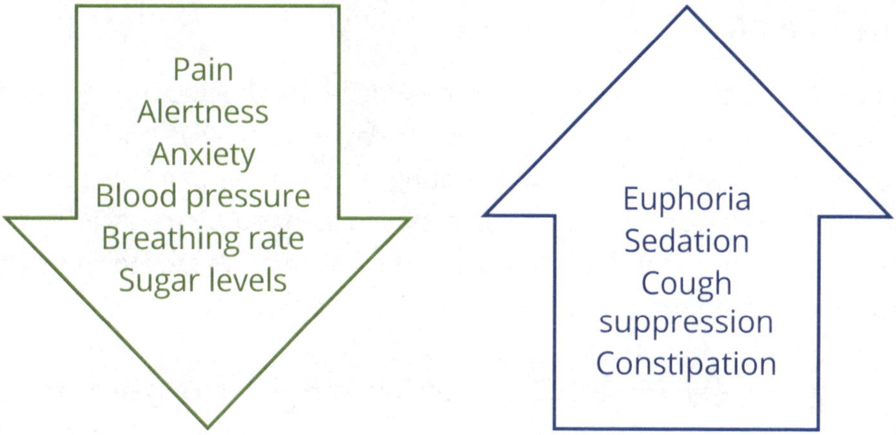

Opioids and Pain

Pain is our body's way of telling us when something is wrong. It is a subjective experience which all of us will experience to some degree throughout our lifetime. Pain affects our mood, mobility and mental health. Our memories, expectations and concerns about the impact of pain can affect our perception of the pain itself. Does this sound familiar? Pain is worse when we are lonely, anxious, low in mood, and when we have few distractions, such as at nighttime, or do not keep our mind and body busy. It is helped by looking after ourselves and keeping occupied, distracted, busy, and active. For many people, it is not a simple case of managing the pain itself, but a complex mix of physical, psychological, social and also economic factors which cannot be 'cured' by popping a pill. Pain can also be helped by non-drug treatments such as electrical stimulation techniques (TENS machines), physiotherapy, acupuncture or psychological approaches such as meditation, mindfulness and Cognitive Behavioural Therapy (CBT).

Acute Pain

Common, everyday pain such as headache, toothache, muscle pain and pain from minor injuries tends to last a relatively short time (a few days or weeks) and is self-limiting because the pain will reduce as the injury heals. This type of short-term pain is often referred to as 'acute' pain and, whilst in some cases the pain may be severe, in other cases treatment may be milder or require no treatment at all.

Opioids are useful for treating acute pain and usually only need to be taken for a period of a few days. They should then be 'tapered down' (reduced) as the pain reduces.

Chronic Pain

Pain that lasts for a longer period of time, perhaps 3 months or more, is known as 'chronic' pain. This persistent pain may be the result of an acute injury or condition but lasts for longer or is more severe than expected. Common types of chronic pain include low back pain and pain caused by arthritis. In many cases of chronic pain, there may be no obvious or visible cause for it, especially for back pain, and it can be affected by many related factors. This means that chronic pain is more difficult to treat than acute pain, and it may be linked to or exacerbated by a number of emotional and social factors, including stress and depression. According to Public Health England, whilst opioids may be effective for acute pain, only a small percentage of chronic pain sufferers find them effective, and those that do find them effective tend to use them at a low dose or intermittently. Long term, high dose opioid use can also cause significant harm, including dependence. It should also be remembered that many codeine-based products contain other ingredients, such as paracetamol. Exceeding the recommended daily dose of paracetamol also can lead to significant health issues including liver damage. In some circumstances, these health issues may have long-term and even fatal outcomes.

Neuropathic Pain

Another type of pain is neuropathic pain which can be of short or long duration. Neuropathic pain can be severe and debilitating. Types of neuropathic pain include pain associated with diabetes, post viral infections (e.g. shingles), multiple sclerosis, sciatica, stroke or limb amputation and post-surgical spine injury.

Cancer Pain

Pain from cancer may straddle all of the above types of pain. Tissue damage or nerve compression may lead to acute pain and some cancer treatments, such as radiotherapy, may lead to neuropathic pain. In addition to the cancer itself, patients may also suffer from other various types of pain. However, for cancer patients facing a terminal diagnosis, treatment with opioids can be effective, especially when the treatment period is short, but the opioids may lose their effectiveness the longer they are used.

A General Overview of the Types of Pain			
	Acute	Chronic	Neuropathic
Severity	Mild to severe	Mild to severe	Mild to severe
Duration	A few days or weeks	More than 3 months	Can be acute but is more often chronic
Usual causes	Tissue/muscle injury, trauma, infections	Occasionally due to unhealed acute injury but often there is no visible cause	Related to nerve-damage or an injury to the central nervous system (affecting the normal signaling processes).
Examples	Headache, toothache, strains, sprains, bone fractures	Lower back pain, arthritis	pain associated with diabetes, post viral infections (e.g. shingles), multiple sclerosis, sciatica, stroke, limb amputation, or post-surgical spine injury.
Are opioids effective?	Yes, for short term use only	Rarely and only short term and at low dose. Non-drug treatments may be more effective	Can be effective for some types but long-term use increases risk of dependence

Opioid-Induced Hyperalgesia (OIH)

Studies have been conducted that demonstrate that the prolonged use of opioids and indeed all types of painkillers can cause increased sensitisation to pain. In other words, the opioids can actually make the pain worse. This is not to be confused with becoming **tolerant** to opioids, which means that over time, the drug loses its effect, and more is needed to obtain the same effect (we will look at this in the next chapter). Opioid-Induced Hyperalgesia means that the opioid *causes* the pain and that pain will worsen as the dose increases. Patients who are diagnosed with OIH are helped by having their opioid reduced or switch to a different type of pain relief.

I hope that you have found this very brief and general overview of opioids and pain useful. As you know, the purpose of this book is to explore opioid addiction and it is therefore important to see the legitimate role opioids should play in the treatment of pain. However, here in the UK, a study published by the reputable medical journal, *The Lancet* revealed that, despite the limitations that opioids have in the management of certain types of pain, prescriptions rose by 34% between 1998 and 2016[†]. Moreover, as well as an increase in the number of prescriptions issued, the average dose also increased. Only 12% of prescriptions for strong opioids were issued for the management of cancer pain, meaning that 88% were prescribed for other acute and chronic pains. Although strong opioids are regularly being used for chronic pain, the National Institute for Health and Clinical Excellence (NICE) makes the following statement in its publication, *'Medicines Opimisation in Chronic Pain 2017'* (updated 2019):

- *There is little evidence that opioids are helpful for chronic pain*

- *A small proportion of people may obtain good pain relief with opioids in the long-term if the dose can be kept low and use is intermittent, but it is difficult to identify these people at the start of treatment*
- *The risk of harm increases substantially at doses above an oral morphine equivalent of 120 mg/day, but there is no increased benefit*
- *Opioids should be discontinued if the person is still in pain despite using opioids, even if no other treatment is available*
- *A detailed assessment of the emotional influences on the person's pain experience is essential for people with chronic pain who also have refractory and disabling symptoms, particularly if they are on high opioid doses*

An alternative to opioids may be found in non-drug treatments which treat the person as a whole. These are often more effective, because stress, depression and poor mental health often go hand in hand with chronic pain. It has long been established that both men and women experiencing social deprivation experience more chronic pain than those better off. Large GP practices in deprived, rural areas in the north of England were associated with prescribing higher doses of opioids[†]. In 2011, 40% of males and 44% of females with the lowest incomes met the *British Pain Society's* criteria for chronic pain, compared with 24% and 30%, respectively, in those with the highest incomes[††].

This leads us nicely into the next chapter which will look more closely at the effect opioids have on us, and the reasons many people may reach for them in an attempt to resolve not only their physical pain but their emotional pain too.

† Curtis H, Croker R et al (2018) *Opioid prescribing trends and geographical variation in England, 1998–2018: a retrospective database* study. The Lancet 2019, 6(2): 140-150 [Online]. Available from https://www.thelancet.com/journals/lanplh/article/PIIS2215-0366(18)30471-1/fulltext [Accessed 11th June 2020]

† † Mordecai L, Reynolds C, Donaldson L, Williams A CdC (2018). *Patterns of regional variation of opioid prescribing in primary care in England:* a retrospective observational study. [Online]. British Journal of General Practice. Available from https://pubmed.ncbi.nlm.nih.gov/29440012/ [Accessed 19th May 2020]

CHAPTER 3
Opioids and Dependence

As we have already said, the relationship between opioids and dependence can be described as the 'perfect storm'. In this chapter, we'll explore exactly what this term means, and lay the foundations for developing our understanding of the causes of opioid dependence and how recovery may be achieved.

We have already seen that endorphins play a key role in managing pain. The word 'endorphin' is taken from the greek word **'endon'** meaning 'within', and the word **morphine**. So 'endorphin' effectively translates as a naturally occurring (endogenous) form of morphine. Endorphins are the body's natural feel good chemicals which are released when we are excited, exercising or in pain. However, endorphins differ from external (exogenous) morphine in that endorphins are not, in themselves, addictive (although this is no doubt due to them only occurring in small amounts).

Endorphins bind to opiate receptors which are mainly found in the brain and spinal cord. Receptors are tiny sites which exist on the cells of the body or brain. There are numerous types of receptors in the body, and once bound to a drug that activates it, they transmit signals to the body or brain. Opiate receptors bind with specific types of drugs, such as opioids and endorphins.

Our natural opioids, the endorphins interact with the reward pathway by binding to the opiate receptors, which then triggers the release of dopamine. When opioids are taken, they also bind to opiate receptors that are concentrated in areas within the reward pathway, and this increases dopamine release. This release of dopamine is a response which becomes **reinforcing**, thus leading to a desire to take more opioids. This is known as **'positive reinforcement'**. Despite their potential to cause dependence, not all users will be affected in this way. The environment (the setting) and the individual's personal makeup (the set) are also extremely important factors. However, as we learnt earlier, the type, quantity and the way the drug is taken are also key factors.

Drugs effects that are enjoyed are more likely to be used repeatedly. Drugs that get to the brain almost immediately (by being smoked, inhaled, snorted or injected) will have a quicker, more intense effect and are more positively reinforcing. They are more likely to cause dependence as the chemical 'reward' is achieved quickly and is more intense. However, this intense and rapid effect does not last long and this means that the user then has to keep repeating the process in order to try to achieve the desired effect. This is known as **'tolerance'**. The faster the onset of effect, the more reinforcing the drug is.

Of course, what goes up, must come down, and the faster the onset of effect, the faster the effects wear off. In fact, the user will very soon find themselves repeating the process, not to achieve the **'reward'** but to ward off the onset of **withdrawal effects.** They will need to continue to use opioids in order to remain 'normal'. This is known as **'negative reinforcement'** as they are continuing to use the drug in order to avoid the negative consequences (withdrawal symptoms) as opposed to attempting to achieve the positive 'feel good' response.

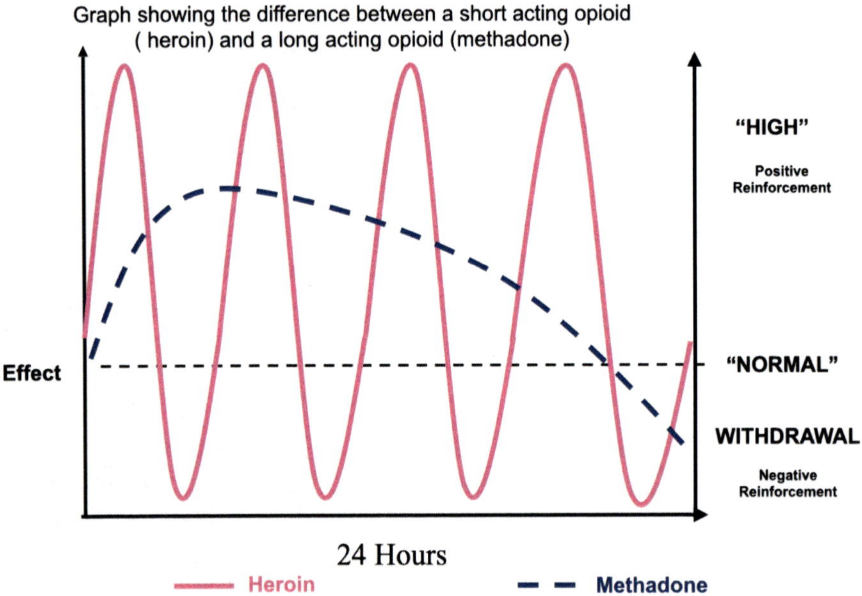

A drug which is taken orally is less reinforcing as it has to be absorbed by the gut and then pass into the blood stream where it travels through the liver. The liver then breaks down (metabolises) the drug, and what remains of the drug continues through the blood stream to the heart, and finally the brain, where it acts on the opioid receptors. The effect of this slower, more gradual uptake results in a delay in the effect of the drug being felt. When the effects are felt, they are not as intense, but will last for longer and wear off more slowly. However, whilst drugs that are taken orally cause less positive reinforcement, they can still lead to both psychological and physical dependence, and the withdrawal effects, though less intense, may last a lot longer. In some cases, the withdrawal can last for weeks or even months.

Interestingly, some drugs, like buprenorphine and naloxone (naloxone is used to reverse an opioid overdose) are broken down so much by the liver that they have little effect if taken orally. This is why these drugs are administered in a way that avoids the liver, i.e. Under the tongue (sublingual), through the skin (transdermal patch), injected in the case of buprenorphine, or injected or inhaled in the case of naloxone.

Some drugs are specifically designed to be absorbed very slowly so that they last even longer and deliver a smoother, more predictable effect. This also makes them less reinforcing. These may be in the form of transdermal patches, e.g. Fentanyl or specially coated tablets e.g. OxyContin®. Once again, it is important to note that these opioids can cause dependence, even when taken as instructed. Moreover, both of these medications have been reported as being misused. For example, by heating the patch to extract the active drug or by crushing the tablets into a powder. These processes mean the drugs can then be smoked, snorted or injected in order to increase their **reward** and **reinforcing** effect.

The *way* a drug is taken helps to explain why heroin is often referred to as one of the most addictive substances. Heroin not only mimics endorphins but is smoked, inhaled (chasing the dragon), snorted or injected. It also explains why medicines such as methadone and buprenorphine, which are used as substitution treatments for addiction to short-acting opioids such as heroin, are often unpopular. Methadone and buprenorphine are both slow onset and long acting opioids which only need to be taken once a day (or sometimes less frequently in the case of buprenorphine). However, whilst they are able to prevent withdrawal symptoms and craving, their slow onset of effect means that they are not psychologically reinforcing enough for some people and this is one of the reasons why people drop out of treatment. We will look at this in more depth in chapter seven.

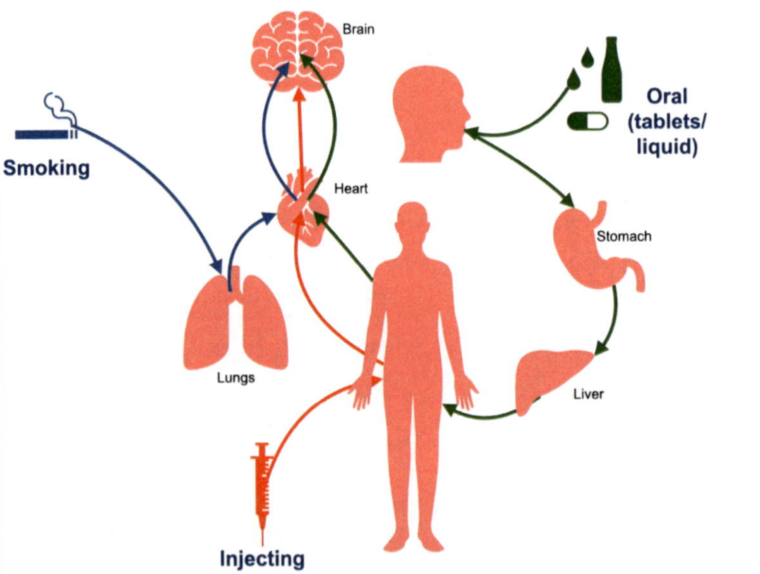

Different Methods of Drug Use

So, to sum up, drugs that are smoked, snorted or injected are considered to be far more reinforcing than drugs that are swallowed. However, regular use of both long and short acting opioids can also lead to **physical and psychological dependence.** Paradoxically, whilst these longer acting drugs are less positively reinforcing, they are often more difficult to stop taking. Stopping may therefore require some form of supported detoxification and careful planning, as it can take weeks or even months for the body to readjust to being without them. We will discuss this in more detail when we look at treatment options.

What is Physical Dependence and Tolerance?

Tolerance

We know that every year millions of people take opioids to manage pain. In most cases, they are able to reduce their dose of opioid as the pain subsides and stop completely without any problems. Many people who take opioids do not actually like the effects they experience from them and are pleased to stop taking them. **Tolerance** is demonstrated when a person either starts to increase the dose or uses the same dose more frequently. This can include topping up with over-the-counter (OTC) medications purchased from a pharmacy or other store, or shortening the time between doses because they are no longer responding to the drug in the way that they used to. In other words, it takes a higher dose of the drug to achieve the same effect that they felt when they started taking the drug. This is because the brain has adapted or become **tolerant** to the presence of the opioids and it is as if the brain is pushing back against the opioids to counteract their effects. We will look at this in more depth in the next chapter but, for now, it is important to note that becoming tolerant to a drug is not the same as being addicted. However, many drugs that are associated with tolerance also have the potential to be addictive.

It is also important to differentiate tolerance from break-through pain caused by worsening of a condition or disease progression; this may also lead to a dose being increased or dosing intervals shortened. Where the opioid is being taken as part of a treatment plan, the healthcare professional should monitor the prescribing closely and look out for signs of dependence such as the patient requesting repeat prescriptions too soon, requesting an increase in dose or topping up with OTC painkillers.

Physical Dependence

With repeated use of opioids, **physical dependence** can occur. Physical dependence occurs when the brain has developed tolerance to the opioid, which results in the appearance of withdrawal symptoms when the drug is reduced or stopped. These symptoms from opioid withdrawal can be extremely severe but are not generally life-threatening - unlike abrupt withdrawal from benzodiazepines and alcohol, which may be fatal if unmanaged. Once again it is important to differentiate between addiction and dependence. Just because someone is **physically dependent** does not mean the person is **addicted.** However, if that person is **addicted,** then **physical dependence** is also generally a factor. An example of this is seen in people being treated with morphine, to manage pain in terminal cancer. There is every likelihood they would experience withdrawal if the morphine was stopped, but their need to use morphine is solely to treat pain and is managed within that context without a compulsion to use it for any other purpose. They are therefore physically dependent but not addicted.

Opioid Withdrawal Symptoms		
Muscle aches	Vomiting	Agitation
Nausea	Diarrhoea	Anxiety
Cramps	Runny nose	Cravings
Sweating	Yawning	Insomnia
Chills	Dilated pupils	Goose-bumps

Psychological Dependence

Psychological dependence presents arguably the greatest challenge when coming to terms with any form of addiction because it can exist independently of physical dependence and is related to neuroadaptation in the brain. The neuroadaptation is thought to be the cause of the psychological dependence, the cravings, tolerance and withdrawal symptoms. To refer back to Zinberg's theory, psychological dependence is closely linked to your 'mind set' which is one of the things that determines how slowly or quickly your brain undergoes neuroadaptation. Psychological dependence occurs from repeatedly stimulating the reward pathway, but it does not need to involve dependence on a drug. Instead, it can involve an activity such as shopping, exercising, gambling or sex – which are known as behavioural addictions.

As we have already discussed, physical dependence upon opioids is the result of a physical change that has happened in response to taking the drug itself. Overcoming physical dependence, though often tough and uncomfortable, can be managed in a planned and controlled way with a beginning, middle and end. Psychological dependence is less about the chemical compound of the drug and more about neuroadaptation that occurs within your brain, which is affected by your personality, emotions and environment. As we have already seen, neuroadaptation refers to the changes in the brain, including your reward pathway, that occur during addiction and which may not be completely reversible. Psychological dependence is far less tangible and harder to define than physical dependence. It is also likely to extend well beyond the duration of that physical dependence because it is about your past, present and future. Recovery from addiction is about understanding what got you to this point, where you are now physically, emotionally and even geographically, where you would wish to be and, most importantly, how you are going to get there. It therefore follows that the groundwork must be laid well in advance of any detox and this preparation will play a key part in your recovery.

CHAPTER 4
Opioids And Emotional Pain

As we know, it is both important and normal for the brain to register pain because experiencing pain is our body's way of telling us that something is wrong- that there is a threat to our well-being. We have discussed the important role that opioids play in managing certain types of physical pain and we also know that prolonged use of opioids can lead to tolerance to the drug's effects as well as dependence, both physical and psychological.

Feelings of stress and anxiety can be due to 'emotional pain', which may relate to past traumas or upsets that still concern us. The symptoms of emotional pain can feel very real. To the person with emotional pain, these symptoms may actually feel as real and uncomfortable as physical pain and it is therefore understandable that a remedy for physical pain is often sought first. When opioids are used to try to manage emotional pain, they are more likely to result in psychological dependence.

Emotional pain may have been lying dormant for years, possibly from childhood, but that emotional pain will have hard-wired that person to respond to stressful situations in a particular way.

Fight, Flight or Freeze - Hyperarousal or the Acute Stress Response

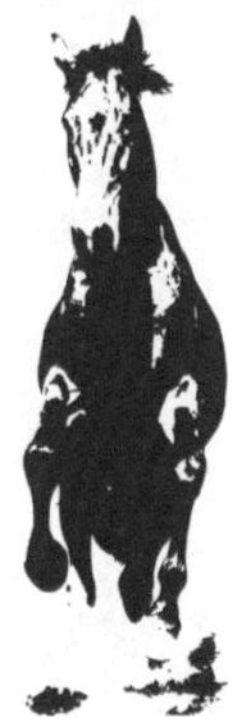

Understanding the 'fight, flight or freeze' response will help to understand why opioids, for many, are the 'drug of choice' for people experiencing emotional pain. In order to understand this better, let us first look at what is widely perceived as the perfect 'fight or flight' animal - The Horse. The survival of the horse through millions of years has depended upon its ability to flee from predators. If fleeing is not an option, the horse is also well equipped to defend itself too by making itself appear bigger and more aggressive by rearing, kicking, striking out and biting. Everything about the horse is designed to protect itself- from its eyes situated on the side of its head giving near 360^0 vision, to its long slender legs, flared nostrils and deep chest cavity.

Human beings also possess the "fight, flight or freeze' response. It is our body's primitive, natural response that prepares us to either stand and fight, or to head to the hills in response to the threat of harm, either real or perceived. When fighting or fleeing is not an option, humans and prey animals resort to 'freezing' to try to conceal their presence. It has been an inherent physiological part of our make up since caveman days but has remained with us into these modern times.

Our Body's Response to a Threat

The amygdala plays a key role in managing our 'fight, flight or freeze' responses. Located in the brain's limbic system, the amygdala, which is also referred to as the 'Fear Centre' or 'Watch Tower', is activated when we express emotional feelings such as sadness, aggression and fear.

When the acute stress response is triggered, our body automatically releases a number of hormones (chemical messengers) into our blood stream which will enable us to either 'fight' or 'flee'. These hormones include adrenaline, cortisol and noradrenaline (also known as norepinephrine). These hormones are often referred to as **'stress hormones'**. One of these stress hormones, noradrenaline, is important for basic daily tasks such as digesting food and even simply getting out of a chair. It is also important for maintaining our brain functions as well as enhancing our levels of concentration and attention. When a threat is imminent, our noradrenaline levels increase. We are now in a state of heightened alertness, which takes priority over normal bodily functions, and a number of changes take place inside our bodies:

- Our blood pressure and heart rate increase to ensure sufficient blood and oxygen reaches our muscles and vital organs, including our brain.
- We release more energy and our pupils dilate to allow our sight and awareness to intensify.
- We may feel nauseous or have the urgent need to be sick or to go to the toilet. This will enable us to 'lighten the load' as we prepare to fight or run.

You body's response to 'Fight and Flight'

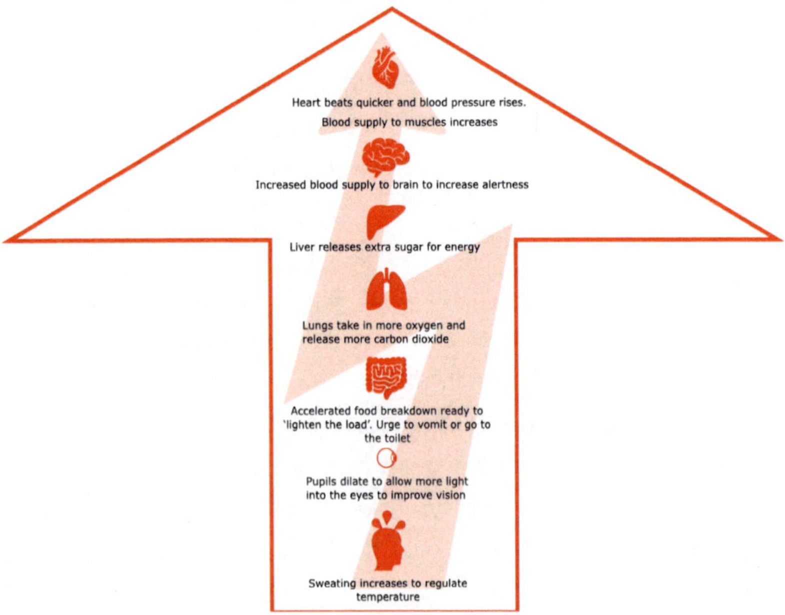

You will have probably already experienced these symptoms at some point in your life. Maybe following a near miss in a car or even during a ride on a roller coaster. You are also likely to have experienced these same symptoms if you have been physically dependent upon opioids and suffered withdrawal effects. We will come back to this later.

What happens when the threat has passed

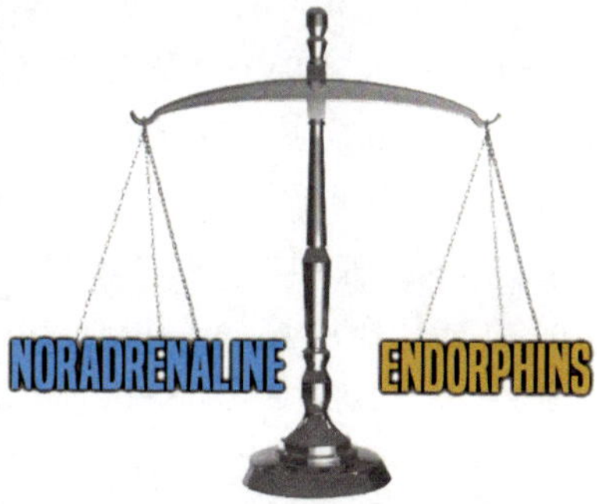

It is not natural for our bodies to exist in this state of heightened alert indefinitely. Once the threat has passed, our body needs to dampen down this state of hyper-arousal and reset the chemical balance. We have already mentioned the key role that noradrenaline plays in the fight or flight response. Noradrenaline has a natural partner, and that partner is endorphins - our body's natural pain killer and feel-good hormone. Noradrenaline and endorphins work together like a set of weighing scales, keeping our bodies finely balanced by working together to ensure that we respond to a threat effectively. When we sense danger, we produce more noradrenaline and fewer endorphins and, when the danger has passed, that process is reversed so that we become balanced again. The fact that that our natural fight and flight response to threat and stress is closely linked to endorphins levels is key to understanding some of the physical and psychological aspects of opioid dependence.

'Fight or flight' in modern times

Looking back through ancient times, most of the threats our ancestors faced were likely to be physical. For example, fear of attack from a predator or another human being.

Modern life contains many stressors, but a certain amount of stress can be a positive thing. For example, feeling stressed can give us that extra edge to get on top of a situation at work or whilst taking part in a competitive activity. However, many modern-day threats which cause harm to our well-being are unseen and more subtle. They may also be entirely psychological. The threat does not even have to be imminent. In fact, this response, which sends various 'stress hormones' coursing through our body, can be triggered even if there is a fear of a threat rather than a threat itself. Our 'fight or flight response' will kick in regardless of whether the threat is physical or psychological. Whilst in this state, we experience heightened alertness and perceive everything around us as a threat to our survival.

However, whilst the *types* of threat we face today have become more sophisticated, our responses to it have not. The 'fight or flight response' has been an invaluable tool enabling us to survive and evolve, yet the fact that it is an automatic response over which we may have little or no control means that, at times it can also be harmful. Most of the threats we face today do not actually require us to physically flee. For example, being late for work or an important event, or having a row with our partner can cause very real levels of stress, but in the main, fleeing, or even fighting, may not be the most appropriated response. Instead, we have to try to manage these stress hormones in a different way by either finding some other methods of expressing ourselves, carrying out an activity to 'let off steam' or by turning emotionally inwards and trying to absorb them.

Chronic stress – Setting the scene for the Perfect Storm

Many of us will experience periods in our life which contain massive amounts of stress. There may be a number of factors going on in our lives or something singularly more serious, such as on-going school or work-based bullying, racial, sexual or cultural prejudices. Similarly, for some of us it will be stressful finding somewhere warm and dry to sleep at night or waiting for an abusive partner or relative to walk through the door. Eventually we subconsciously begin to see everything and everyone as a threat and what may normally feel like a minor irritation, such as someone being upset with you, losing your keys or another road user pulling out in front of you, can be blown out of all proportion. For many people who become addicted to drugs, this chronic stress began in childhood. Experiencing directly or indirectly some form of trauma or several types of trauma means that you are far more likely to get into addiction. This trauma could relate to physical, sexual or psychological abuse (including physical and emotional neglect) and may have been buried for years, decades even. Evidence suggests that the younger the child and the longer the duration of the trauma, the greater the challenge for the individual to recover. Trauma is not just confined to people living in poorer communities. Children who have been raised in privileged environments are also commonly victims of all types of abuse, including neglect. Poverty is not a guarantee of bad parenting and wealth is not a guarantee of good parenting. Whilst many physical needs may be met in a wealthy or comfortable family, an ability to meet the emotional needs of children may be absent. Individuals who have experienced such emotional pain may revert to 'fight or flight' mode at the slightest provocation or potential threat, as this default setting may have been hardwired to 'survival mode' from a very young age. It is important to say at this point that, if the 'hard-wiring' was done at a very young age, this stress response will have been set by an unsophisticated, undeveloped child's brain. This means that stressors or threats experienced by the adult will still be managed by this childhood response, regardless of how rational the adult's brain is in comparison. In these situations, psychotherapy or other treatment for trauma is likely to be required in order to effectively unlock this childhood reaction to stress and reset the fight or flight response to allow stress to be managed by the adult brain i.e. in a more rational, sophisticated way.

Extended periods of stress, at whatever age, will result in an overall increase in the 'stress hormone' noradrenaline and a reduction in the 'feel good hormone', endorphin, putting us in permanent 'fight or flight' mode. In addition, people experiencing chronic stress will have fewer opiate receptors, as they have far fewer endorphins to occupy them. For many people, that natural 'feeling of well-being' produced by endorphins becomes either rare or non-existent. They will therefore find it more difficult to visualise positive outcomes and to make balanced, rational decisions. This will inevitably result in a further increase in stress and anxiety. This downward spiral can then become a self-fulfilling prophecy.

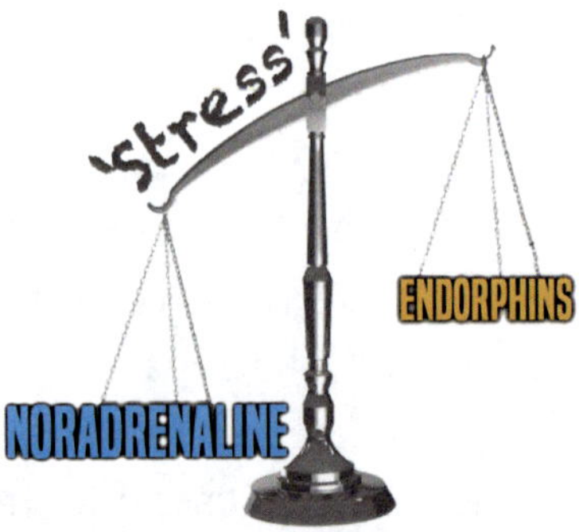

The NHS has provided this simple, yet effective table to identify stress

Symptoms of Stress www.nhs.uk/conditions/stress-anxiety-depression/understanding-stress/			
How you may feel emotionally	How you may feel mentally	How you may feel physically	How you may behave
Overwhelmed	Lacking in self-esteem	Headaches	Drinking alcohol or smoking more
Irritable and "wound up"	Racing thoughts	muscle tension or pain	Snapping at people
Anxious or fearful	Constantly worrying	Dizziness	Avoiding things or people you are having problems with
	Difficulty concentrating	Sleep problems	
		Feeling tired all the time	
		Eating too much or too little	

Chronic Stress- Food for thought

Everyone's experience of life and ability to cope with certain aspects of it is entirely individual. No two people will experience the exact same situation and feel and respond to it in exactly the same way. This is what makes recognising, managing and treating chronic stress such a challenge, because until you have actually walked in someone's shoes you cannot truly experience what they are going through. Chronic stress does not have to involve headline grabbing situations such as the Jimmy Saville scandal or even clearly identifiable scenarios which have a defined label, such as bullying, sexual, racial or religious discrimination. In fact, trying to compare your situation with that of others can only exacerbate things by adding a sense of guilt, shame, blame and weakness. It is too easy to believe that there are so many people who seem to cope better than you despite appearing to have suffered far worse than you. We often feel that our difficulty coping is due to our perception of our own lack of inner strength or even selfishness. In fact, our ability to cope has a lot to do with our experiences of life as a child, including how well our parents could read us, and the stresses and traumas we had. We may indeed have become chronically stressed as a child through things that were entirely outside of our control. Chronic stress can also creep up on you even when everything around you appears to be fine, as there can be underlying stressors which are pressing on your mental well-being. These stressors could be external, maybe a lack of support or recognition at work, financial worries or a difficult relationship with a partner, friend or family member. They could be internal, such as low self-esteem, self-doubt, helplessness or just a feeling of loneliness and isolation often made worse by the feelings of guilt mentioned previously.

Whatever the reason, recovery from this situation will often require drastic changes to your life before things have a chance of improving.

Opioids and Chronic Stress- The Perfect Storm

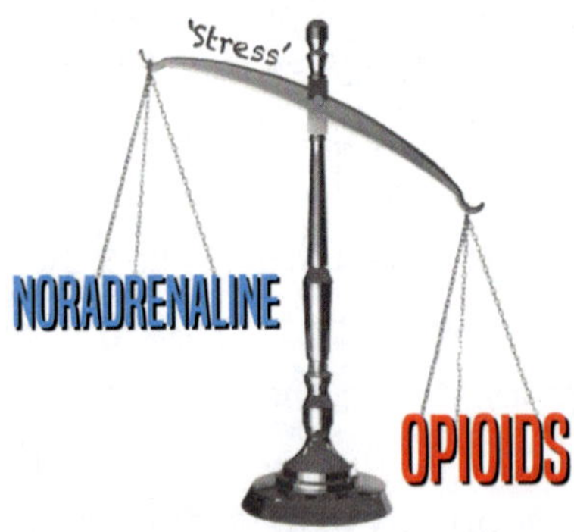

Opioids we use, whether illicit or prescribed, act like exogenous endorphins, except that we do not produce them naturally. When we first take opioids, they take on the role of endorphins. They flood the existing opioid receptors and *push back* the noradrenaline levels. What does this mean to the person suffering from chronic stress or emotional pain? Well for the first time in probably a very long time, the fight or flight sensation will subside and be replaced by a feeling of well-being or euphoria. People often describe their early use of opioids as like being wrapped in a warm blanket or cotton wool. Emotional pain and certain types of physical pain will also be reduced and so overall, the experience for that individual will be a positive one and one which they will wish to repeat. In addition to the feelings of well-being, they will also experience a number of physical effects. Heart rate and blood pressure will fall, and breathing will also be suppressed.

Your body's response to opioid administration

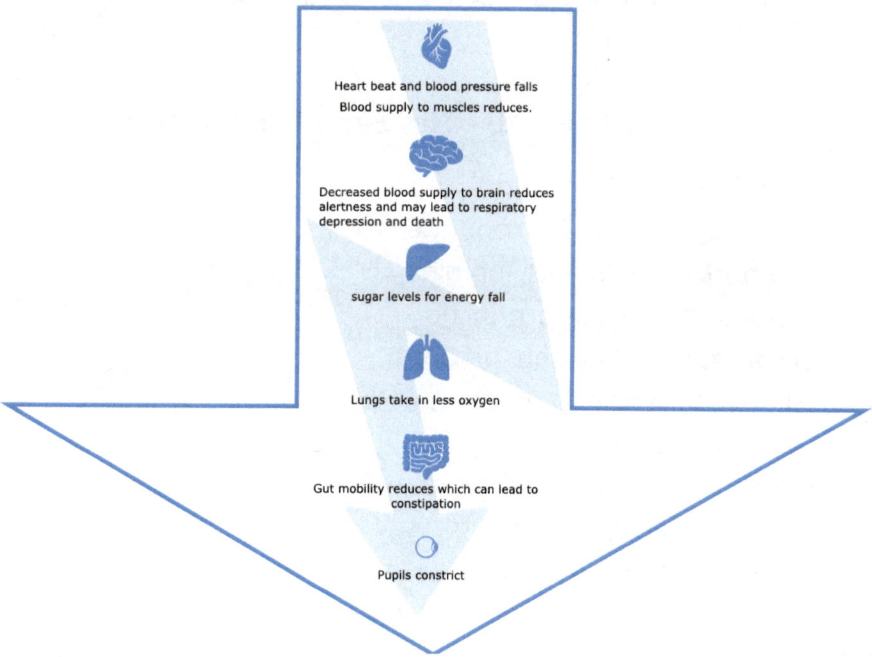

Repeating the experience can be risky, as it can lead to a potentially fatal overdose caused by respiratory depression, especially for people who have just started using opioids for the first time. It can also be dangerous for individuals who have just started taking opioids again after a break as they will have lost their ***tolerance*** to the effects of opioids. The risks of a fatal overdose are further increased if opioids are taken with other drugs that can also have a suppressant effect on breathing, such as alcohol and benzodiazepines (diazepam etc). At this point it is also worth remembering what we have learnt about positive reinforcement. We know that the opioids will act like endorphins and help to reduce noradrenaline and, as a result, stress or emotional pain. This effect will be ***positively reinforcing***. In addition, this reinforcement can be further enhanced by using a route by which the opioid gets to the brain quicker, which increase the speed and intensity of the effect.

Continued use of opioids- The Eye of the Storm

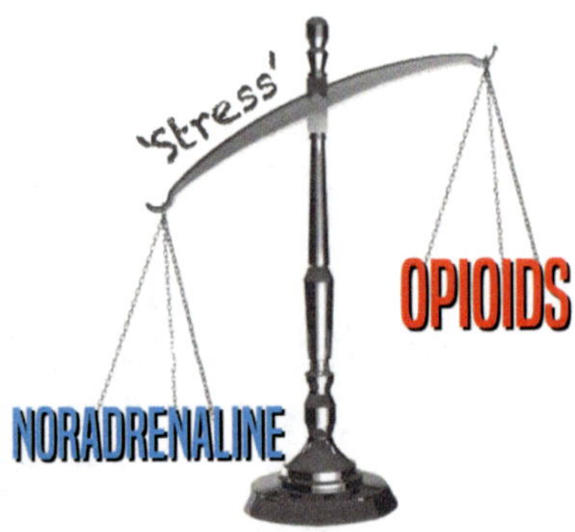

If you continue to take opioids, your levels of noradrenaline will continue to be suppressed. In fact, opioids actually shut down the production of noradrenaline. For the person who is experiencing emotional pain, this will feel like a good thing, as the amount of noradrenaline you produce naturally due to the stress will be far higher than someone who is not stressed. The opioids will occupy the opiate receptors in your brain and effectively do the job endorphins should be doing. There are, however, a couple of consequences to this situation. Firstly, your brain will produce even fewer of its natural endorphins. This happens because when the receptors are already occupied by the opioids, this tells the brain to produce fewer endorphins. Secondly, as the effects of the opioids begin to wear off, the brain will respond by increasing the amount of noradrenaline it produces. You are, after all, suffering from stress, the cause of which has not yet been addressed. The presence of the opioids is interfering with your brain's default setting which is 'fight or flight', and for this you will need more noradrenaline.

So, the brain responds by increasing production of noradrenaline so that your levels are back to 'normal' (normal for you) again, only now your stress may actually have increased because you need to acquire and use opioids regularly - possibly illicitly!

This situation is likely to prompt you to take even more opioids to try to regain the positive feelings you originally experienced, and to reduce the feelings of stress and, possibly withdrawal. If you are taking something that is 'short acting', like heroin, then you will need to repeat this process several times a day. Remember, the route by which a drug is taken (smoking or injecting) will affect the level of positive reinforcement experienced in the early days and the more reinforcing it is, the harder it will push you to seek more drugs. If this cycle is allowed to continue, tolerance will develop, and you will no longer experience the **reward** but instead you will be experiencing unpleasant **withdrawal symptoms** as each dose wears off. For those individuals who are using illicit drugs or using their prescription in an unauthorised way, they are likely to experience the additional stress of sourcing a regular supply and the negative consequences legally, financially and personally that go with it. By now, they may have become physically and psychologically dependent upon opioids and are faced with a number of very serious and challenging options. In short, the opioids, which initially appeared to make things better have now in fact made life a lot worse.

CHAPTER 5
The Opioid Withdrawal Syndrome

We now understand that emotional pain and the effect opioids have on our body combine to produce the ideal recipe for the perfect storm. After continued use of opioids, our brain fights back. It does this in order to protect us by increasing our stress hormones and preparing us again for the fight or flight response. The more opioids we take, the more stress hormones we produce when the opioids start to wear off. After a while, we will have also become tolerant to the effects of the opioids and physically and psychologically dependent upon them too. Our life will have has become a daily cycle of obtaining, taking and recovering from opioids. There are few positives now, almost all negatives, and our lifestyle has become even more stressed than it was before. We may feel trapped in needing to continue to use opioids to feel okay, but hardly getting any positive benefit from them. So, what can be done? Just as it is important to understand what happens in our brain when we use opioids, we now need to look at what happens when we stop. By understanding this, we can predict and prepare for what is to come and that, in itself, will make the whole process more manageable. However, physical withdrawal is only part of the story. We also need to develop robust strategies for managing the psychological aspects of opioid dependence. This is likely to be the greatest challenge, requiring lots of support, especially after the physical withdrawal period has been completed. For many, detoxification from opioids is like lifting the lid on Pandora's box; all kinds of memories are likely to come to the surface, sometimes for the first time in years. It is vital that you put a range of safety nets in place before you begin the detoxification process. If this does not happen, a relapse will be much more likely to take place, and you will find it even more difficult to 'lift the lid' in the future.

The Opioid Withdrawal Syndrome (OWS)

The first thing to understand about the OWS is that it is not, in itself, life-threatening in those who are otherwise healthy. Although the symptoms may be extremely unpleasant, they will not kill you, and they *will* pass.

Now, before we look at what happens in the brain when opioids are suddenly stopped, let us have a quick recap:

Noradrenaline is a stress hormone that is essential for maintaining normal body and brain function. It has a natural partner called endorphins. Endorphins are 'feel good' chemicals naturally produced by the brain when the body experiences pain or stress. They are also known as the 'natural' opiates of the body.

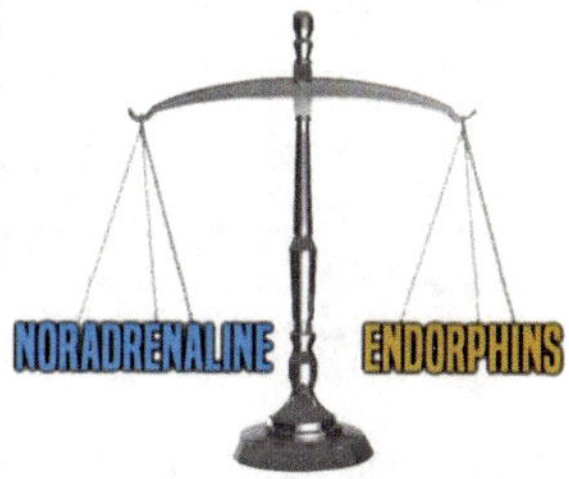

Chronic stress can cause high levels of noradrenaline, and high levels of noradrenaline can cause stress.

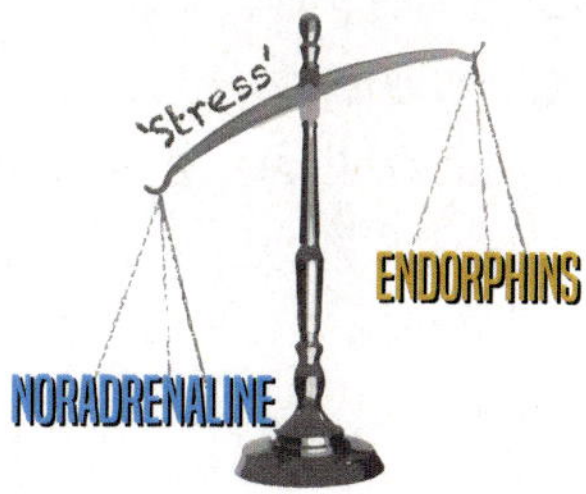

Opioids are like endorphins, and their action causes an upset between the natural balance of endorphins and noradrenaline, resulting in a temporary reduction of noradrenaline and therefore reducing stress. As the opioids start to wear off, more noradrenaline is therefore produced to bring things back into balance.

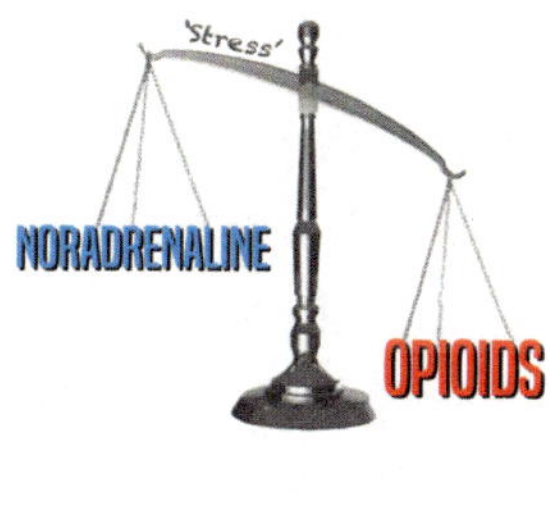

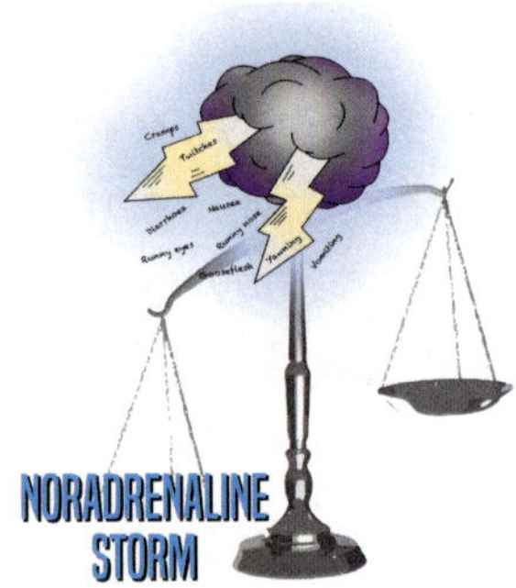

However, after a period of prolonged use, when the opioids are stopped suddenly, the noradrenaline is no longer suppressed, but the brain continues to produce it. This leads to a phenomenon called the 'noradrenaline storm', which is caused by an excessive amount of noradrenaline, and is responsible for most of the symptoms of opioid withdrawal. Abrupt opioid withdrawal resembles a severe bout of 'flu and is also often referred to as 'cold turkey' because one of the signs is goose bumps on the skin ('goose flesh') which resemble the skin of a plucked refrigerated turkey.

How severe will the storm be?

The speed of onset, severity and duration of the OWS will depend upon both the *quantity and type* of opioids that have been taken, as well as the *way* they have been taken. So, just as someone who injects heroin will get a more rapid, intense but short-lived response, the OWS will likewise be more rapid, intense but short-lived.

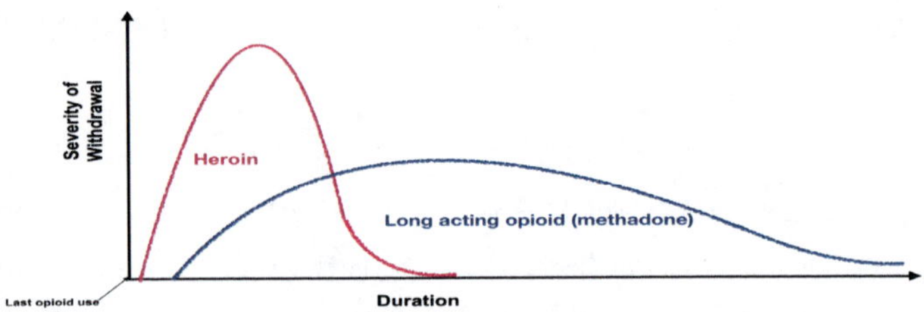

Likewise, someone who has been taking a long-acting opioid, such as methadone, will experience a slower onset of OWS, but the symptoms will go on for longer.

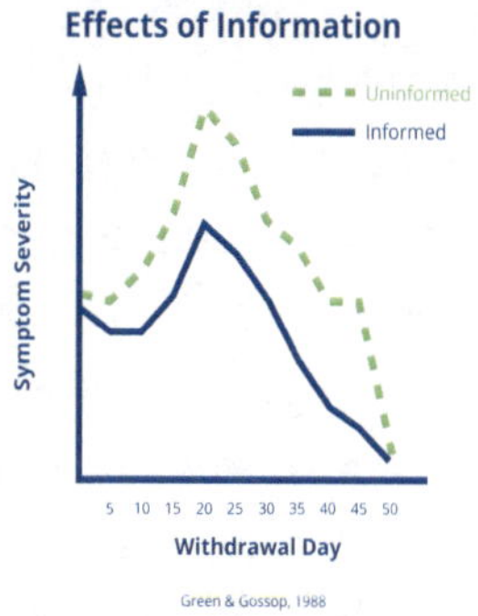

It is extremely helpful to learn as much as you can about the withdrawal process and what to expect, because this will have a positive effect on your symptoms. Each situation and person are different, and this book will hopefully help you to make informed choices about your own experience.

We will look more closely at medical strategies for managing opioid dependence, including detoxification, in the next chapter, but it is important to understand that no detoxification is going to be symptom-free. There is no way of coming off opioids without experiencing some opioid withdrawal symptoms – there is "no gain without pain". There are, however, various medications available, many over-the-counter, that can help deal with specific troublesome symptoms as shown in the following table:

Symptom	Medication	Availability
Diarrhoea	Loperamide hydrochloride e.g Imodium	GSL
Nausea, vomiting, may also be useful for stomach cramps	Metoclopramide e.g Maxalon Prochlorperazine e.g Buccastem	POM POM
Stomach cramps	Mebeverine e.g Colofac	POM
Muscular pains and headaches	Paracetamol, ibuprofen, aspirin	GSL

Key:
GSL= General Sales List (GSL). Available in general retail outlets. A pharmacist does not need to be present to sell it to you. POM = Prescription Only Medicine

Symptoms such as agitation, anxiety and sleeplessness may require medications such as diazepam or zopiclone, but these medications can also cause dependence and should be used with caution. If they are needed, they should only be prescribed for a short period of time, as part of the withdrawal process. Other approaches which do not involve medication, such as meditation and mindfulness, are worth exploring as they teach you skills which will help you to not only manage your moods and feelings now and in the future, but also to understand your past feelings and emotions.

It is helpful to remember that, although withdrawal symptoms are uncomfortable, their progress is usually predictable, with a beginning, middle and end, especially if a good amount of effort has been put into preparation for it. However, some drugs, including opioids in a proportion of people, can lead to prolonged or protracted withdrawal, lasting for months and sometimes longer. People who have consumed a large amount of a drug over a long period of time, or who have psychological issues, are more likely to experience this. These symptoms are generally mood-related, such as sleep disturbances, anxiety, depression, irritability and fatigue but they may also be physical, including aches and pains. Either way, these protracted symptoms may feel as intense as the symptoms experienced during the early stages of withdrawal and result in a relapse to opioid use in an attempt to stop the discomfort.

The Mountain and the Molehill

We have now looked at the physical aspects of opioid withdrawal, and what happens in our brain as well as the rest of our body. However, we know that for people who are both physically and psychologically dependent, this is only part of the story. Anyone who is psychologically dependent and wishing or needing to stop taking opioids, who believes that all they need to do is manage the physical symptoms of withdrawal, is setting themselves up to fail.

"There is a widely held, simplistic belief amongst both treatment providers and those living with addiction, that in order to overcome dependence on opioids, all someone had to do was undergo a short period of detoxification and they would be 'cured'. The common but simplistic perception of many people, including healthcare professionals and the general public, is that detox from opiates is over in about a couple of weeks – you just have to get over the mountain of withdrawal symptoms to be safe on the other side. You may slip back during the detoxification if your symptoms are too severe, but if you can get over to the other side, you will generally be safe. The idea is that when someone is opioid dependent, the changes in the brain that occur during dependence have an enormous impact on their behaviour i.e. they continue to seek drugs. However, once they have decided to detox, they simply have to get over the mountain of detoxification symptoms, so they are no longer dependent, and can once again be free to control their own life. Once they are in the land of the drug free, they can choose to remain there or, if they so choose, decide to walk around the mountain by using drugs again, and again developing dependence. The fact that the ground level is the same on both sides of the mountain indicates that this is a free choice, and that there is no significant predisposition that means an abstinent individual is any more likely to take up using drugs again than anyone else. This model is more or less true if only the more obvious physical aspects of withdrawal are considered important."

Dr Fergus Law, MBChB, BSc, FRCPsych

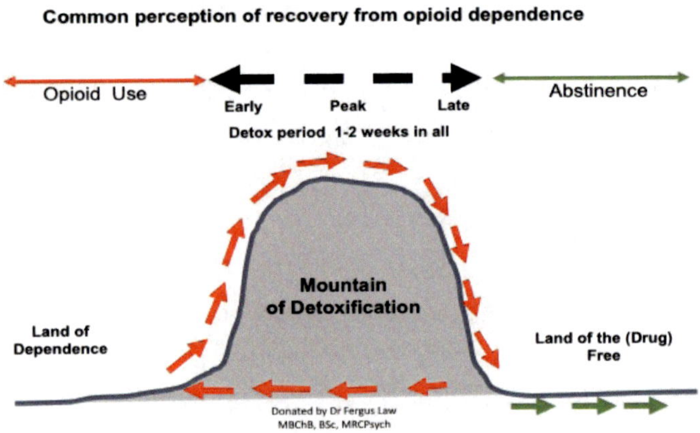

However, the reality is somewhat different. As the author Mark Twain famously said in reference to his smoking addiction, 'giving up (smoking) is easy, I've done it hundreds of times!'. So instead of the detox being the mountain, it is in fact sustaining recovery and maintaining abstinence that is the mountain. The physical withdrawal period is, by comparison, a molehill.

"The research evidence however supports a more complicated view – there are more subtle physical and psychological changes that have a massive impact during dependence and abstinence. The acute detoxification is merely a transitional state between dependence and early abstinence (during which protracted withdrawal symptoms occur) which ultimately leads to the more secure state of late abstinence. Indeed, the acute detox by comparison is simply a small molehill which pales into insignificance compared to the enormous and prolonged effort that is required to remain abstinent. Indeed, it may take 4-7 years for the protracted withdrawal symptoms to resolve and for someone to develop normal physiology, and normal levels of self-esteem and anxiety. It is clear that a person who remains abstinent needs continued encouragement and should be

given an enormous amount of respect and support. Even when they have succeeded in getting over this mountain, they still have a predisposition to relapse, as indicated by the land being higher on that side – physical predispositions do remain, and even though conditioned responses may have been extinguished, these responses can be reactivated under certain conditions. Indeed, relapse can happen very rapidly, and they may quickly slip back to the land of dependence. The implication is that someone who has achieved abstinence needs to remain alert and on guard even after many years of abstinence."

Dr Fergus Law MBChB, BSc, FRCPsych

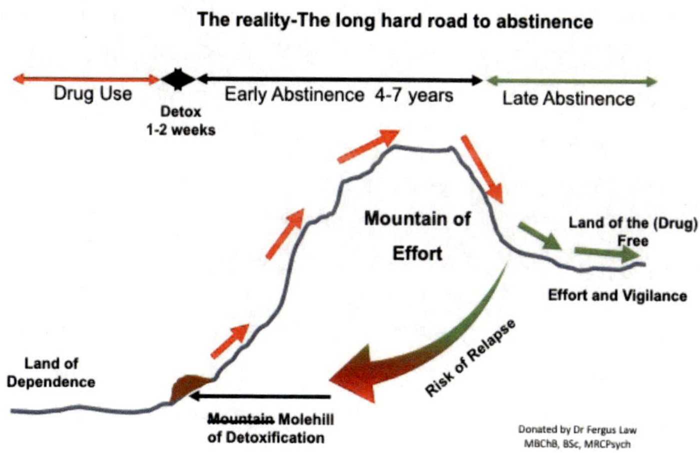

Very few people who are physically and psychologically dependent are able to achieve long term abstinence on the first attempt. Instead, they may make multiple attempts, learning new things with every attempt, before achieving sustained abstinence. However, each unsuccessful attempt should not be viewed as a failure. You may recall the 'driving test' analogy I described at the start of this book: "*learning to drive comes a lot easier for some than for others. No two*

experiences are the same, but the key thing to remember is that nearly everyone passes their test at some point and goes on to become a safe and competent driver".

It is true that a lot can be learnt from each so-called 'failed attempt'. With something as complex as opioid dependence, which crosses every strand of our life, each attempt will not take place in a vacuum. Life moves on, people's priorities, outlook on life and physical and mental health will continue to alter over time. Research, including that carried out by the Recovery Research Institute, has shown that, for many people, the things that ultimately help them to succeed are a combination of being sick and tired of the lifestyle, being able to 'move away' from their old life, both physically and psychologically and actively building new emotional or spiritual support networks for themselves. For more information, you can visit the Recovery Research Institute website at www.recoveryanswers.org.

Opioids and sleep

We all need sleep, but the amount of sleep we need will vary between individuals and will also depend on our age and level of activity. A typical adult generally requires between seven and eight hours of sleep per night

Quality, as well as quantity of sleep, is important in ensuring our body and mind are healthy. We tend to think of sleep as a time when our bodies and mind shut down, but actually this is when our body actively restores, rejuvenates and repairs itself. Sleep is an active time for our mind too, as it is a time when we process events and thoughts and organises them in our memory banks. A good sleep pattern involves consistent, healthy routines that allow us, regardless of our age, to achieve the right balance in terms of quality and quantity.

Sleep has five different stages which are divided into REM (Rapid Eye Movement) and Non-REM sleep, each with its own vital role. When we sleep at night, we generally cycle through these stages 2 or 3 times, and also wake up several times but rarely remember this.

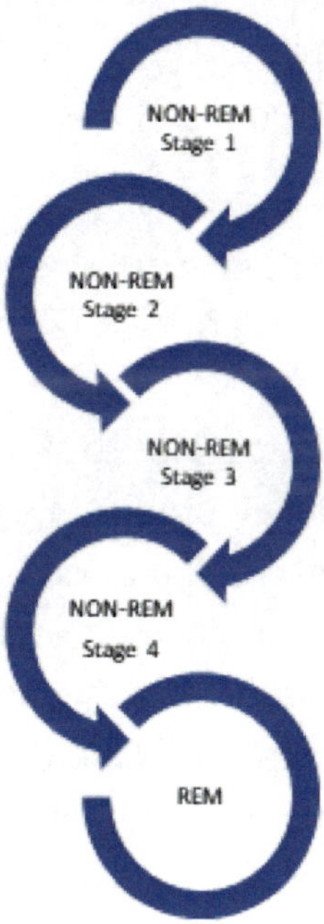

1.Transition between awake and sleep

2. Light sleep. Our breathing slows, muscles relax and heart rate drops

3-4 Deep sleep. We restore, rejuvenate and repair

REM Usually occurs around 90 minutes after falling asleep and lasts about 1 hour. This is our dreaming sleep where we process, store and learn

What causes sleep problems?

- Physical - The normal effects of aging (we need less sleep as we get older). Illness or conditions such as pain, restless legs, sleep apnoea, asthma. Lifestyle, including shift working and jet lag
- Psychological - Anxiety and depression, grief, stress and Post Traumatic Stress Disorder. This often means that we have difficulty going to sleep, awake more in the night, and awake early and are unable to get back to sleep. Vigilance, such as listening out for young children, for any potential threat, or being 'on call'
- Pharmacological – The effects of medications or drugs e.g. opioids, alcohol, caffeine etc or withdrawal from drugs

Many people suffering from long-term chronic pain use opioids to take away pain and stop their sleep being disrupted. However, opioids also disrupt our sleep patterns, in particular blocking both REM and deep sleep. In addition, opioids are known to affect our breathing and can cause 'sleep apnoea' (which is when your breathing stops and starts while you sleep) which can result in snoring, gasping for air, dry mouth, awaking, feeling tired, and having a headache in the morning.

Insomnia is also a leading cause of relapse for people withdrawing from opioids, as sleep disruption can be severe and prolonged following detoxification from any opioid. These disturbances include an inability to sleep, restlessness, delayed sleep latency (this is the time it takes to fall asleep), prolonged periods of wakefulness, vivid dreams and not feeling refreshed by sleep. People will often feel that they have not slept at all, because the sleep they do get is of a poor quality – mainly stage 1 and 2 sleep. Insomnia is most severe during the peak of withdrawals, and sleep medication (hypnotics) may be helpful at this stage but has limited effect. Psychological approaches are the preferred treatment during mild to moderate insomnia, and for chronic insomnia, to reduce the risk of physical or psychological dependence on hypnotics. Hypnotics are best used when insomnia is severe, and when the insomnia lasts for a defined period of time, as can occur during opiate withdrawal. They are not recommended for longer than 2-4 weeks, as specified in their licence.

Good sleep habits

Establishing good sleep habits may involve developing a routine and regular timetable of activities and sticking to it. You should improve your surroundings to promote sleep. For example, try to use fresh bedding, and make sure your room is not too hot or too cold. Use ear plugs to block out unnecessary noise and consider listening to relaxation or meditation recordings – there are plenty of free or inexpensive online resources available to use as you are winding down before going to bed. Using essential oils can also help promote relaxation, in particular lavender, rose and basil. The return of a natural sleep pattern does not happen overnight but may take several weeks or months, so a lot of patience may be required. The following tips can help to achieve a good night's sleep:

Overcoming sleep problems- Dos and Don'ts

DOs	DONTs
Do have a bedtime routine to wind down; go up to bed and get up at a regular time	Don't worry about not getting enough sleep
Do get out of bed if you are unable to fall asleep within 30 minutes or so	Don't watch TV or do anything in bed other than sleep and sex
Do exercises regularly during the day but avoid doing so in the evenings	Don't eat sugary foods, smoke cigarettes or drink caffeine drinks before going to bed
Do make sure your bedroom is comfortable	Don't drink alcohol close to bedtime
Do keep a sleep diary. You probably are sleeping more than you think you are	Don't take naps in the daytime

Opioid Overdose

We have spent a fair bit of time looking at the balancing act that is constantly taking place in our brains between opioids, endorphins and our stress hormones, and what happens when opioids are reduced or stopped suddenly. But what happens when the amount of opioid in your body tips the scales to the point of overdose?

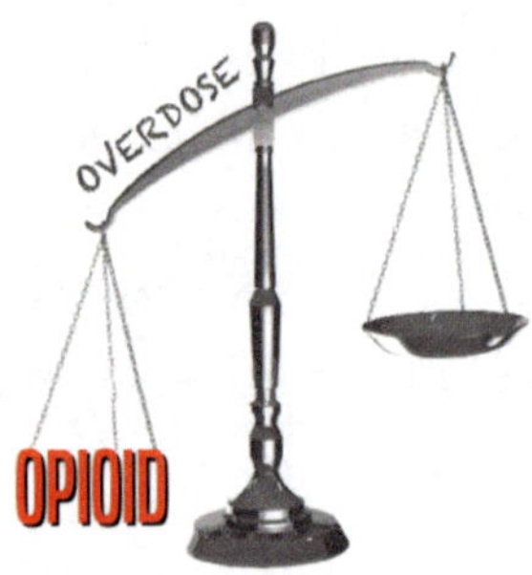

To begin with, here are some alarming facts:

- 34% of all recorded drug overdoses in Europe occur in the United Kingdom
- According to the Office of National Statistics, the number of drug-related deaths (DRDs) in England and Wales is increasing and at least 54% of DRDs involved opioids
- The death rate of opioid users is six times higher than that of the general population
- You are 40 times more likely to die of a fatal overdose in the first 2 weeks of leaving a secure or protective environment (e.g. a prison or hospital) where access to opioids is restricted or prohibited
- Using other substances, such as alcohol and benzodiazepines increase the risk of overdose
- The risk of overdose increases if opioids are injected (rather than smoked)

Injecting drugs also puts people at risk of other life-threatening consequences, especially if they share needles with others. These risks include contracting bacterial infections such as endocarditis (which is an infection of the lining of the heart), tuberculosis, and viral infections, such as HIV and hepatitis B and C. Studies have shown that between 70-90% of injecting drug users are hepatitis C positive.

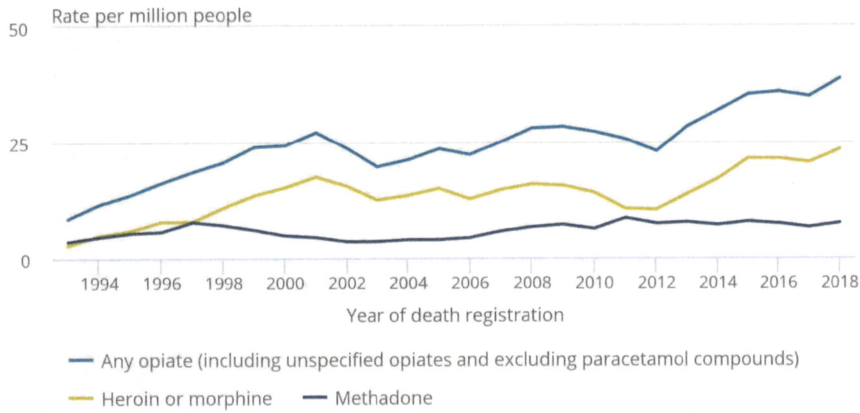

What causes an opioid overdose and why are they so dangerous?

In chapter three, we looked at physical and psychological dependence and the role **tolerance** plays in this. Remember, tolerance means that the brain has adapted to the presence of opioids, so that more opioids are needed to produce the same effect.

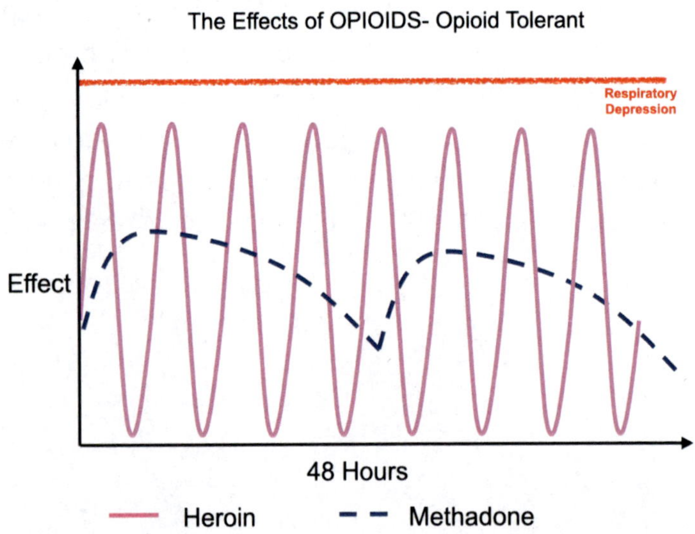

However, if the opioid user increases the dose of opioid or takes other substances such as alcohol or benzodiazepines, the risk of overdose increases. Likewise, the risk of overdose increases after a period of abstinence, which is why the risks are so great for people who start to use opioids again after spending time away from opioids e.g. following a detoxification or leaving a prison or hospital setting. Too often, the individual will return to using opioids at the same dose as they used before they stopped. Injecting opioids also increases the risk because in addition to the more rapid and intense response, it is also often impossible to know exactly what you are actually injecting in terms of strength and quantity of the opioid.

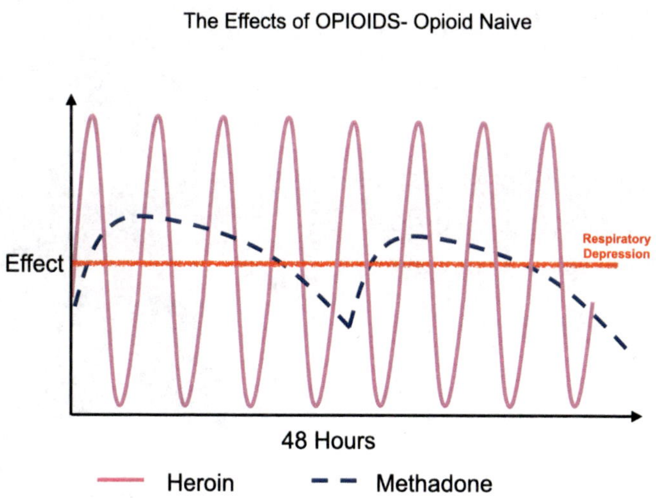

What causes an opioid overdose?

Opioids effect the part of the brain which regulates breathing. Opioids in high doses can reduce your rate and depth of breathing, which leads to respiratory depression. Respiratory depression is the main cause of an opioid overdose and is potentially life-threatening. It is, in fact, the cause of most fatalities and is also more likely to affect people with poor lung function such as smokers and those with COPD, asthma and chronic bronchitis. Respiratory depression can occur very quickly, but it can also take a while, perhaps hours, to build up and can also occur during sleep.

The signs of an overdose include:

- No response to noise (where you 'shout' at the suspected overdose casualty and get no response).
- No response to touch (shoulder shake).
- Loss of consciousness i.e. the suspected overdose casualty cannot be woken.
- Breathing problems
- Slow/shallow or infrequent breaths
- Snoring/rasping sounds
- Not breathing at all
- Bluish, greyish or pale skin
- Bluish tinge to lips, tip of nose, eye bags, fingertips or nails

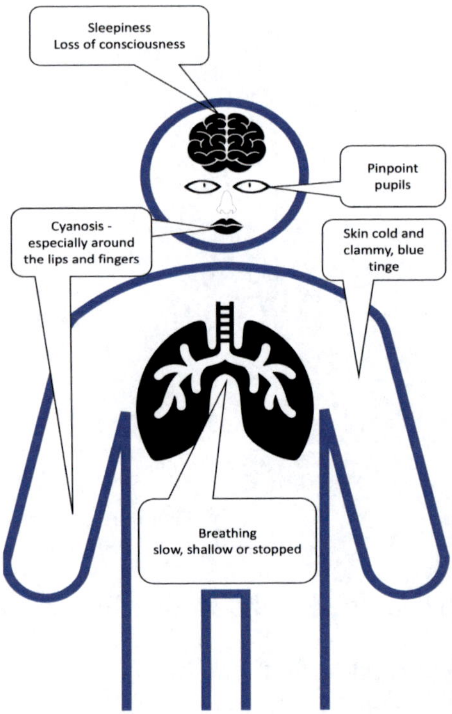

It is important to note that, whilst some overdoses are intentional, others are an avoidable consequence of taking opioids and, in many cases, are reversible providing certain actions are taken promptly. These actions include:

- Call 999 immediately and asking for an ambulance, telling the operator that the casualty is unconscious and explaining whether or not they are breathing.
- Gently open the mouth and look inside, checking for anything that is blocking the airway.
- Open their airway by gently tilting their head back and opening their mouth.
- Look, listen and feel for signs of breathing for no more than 10 seconds.

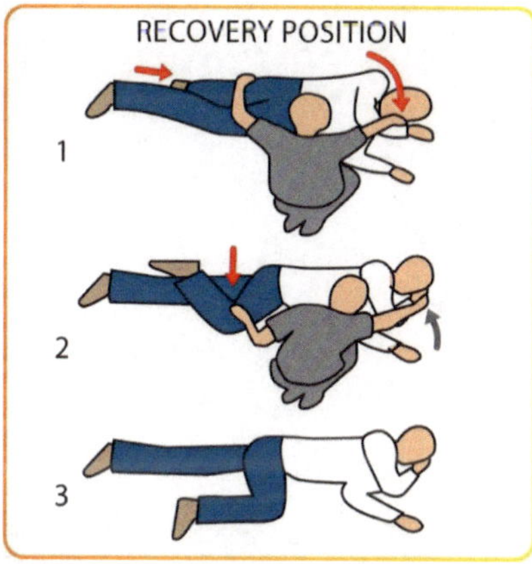

- Move the casualty so that they are lying in the recovery position.
- 6. Follow any other instructions you get from the 999 operator until the ambulance arrives.
- Administer naloxone, which is a 'rescue medication' used to reverse opioid overdoses. We will cover this in the next chapter

We have now looked at what happens to our body and mind when we stop using opioids, as well as when we take too many. In the next couple of chapters, we will explore the most common treatment approaches which are adopted for people who are opioid dependent. This includes opioid substitution treatments (OST), relapse prevention and reversal of overdose. We will outline how each medication works, as well as unpicking the rationale for the various approaches. It is important to appreciate that no treatment can work in isolation. Psychological support needs to be wrapped around any medical intervention in order to deliver a successful outcome. We may also need to accept that it may take several attempts, over a number of months or years for our goals to be reached BUT, most importantly, they CAN be reached!

CHAPTER 6
Starting the Recovery Journey

We have reached a point in the book where we can now prepare for the start of the journey to recovery from opioid dependence. This will involve setting your individual goals, both short term and long term. For example, you may feel that you are committed to a life free from opioids but for now, there are too many issues in the here and now that are taking your energy. Your goal may even be to continue to use opioids for the foreseeable future, but that you would like to manage the harm they are causing to your physical or emotional health. Whatever your goal is, it is highly likely that, for now at least, this will involve you continuing to take opioids, albeit in the short term. In that case, it is good to have a better understanding of the most commonly used pharmaceutical approaches to treating opioid dependence, so that you can be more prepared and make the right decisions for you. Always remember that no treatment option is a panacea; they all have their strengths and weaknesses and that medications should only be viewed as a crutch to help you along the road. An over-reliance on any medication is an easy trap to fall into; after all, seeking a 'pill for very ill' may be what got you into this situation in the first place.

To put this into context further, you should now be able to fully appreciate the physical, emotional, social and psychological ingredients that make up addiction. The physical, or 'drug' part of addiction is probably the easiest aspect to understand and manage, as illustrated by the 'mountain and molehill' analogy. That is not to say that you will not be presented with challenges as you begin to stabilise, reduce and ultimately terminate your use of opioids, but working on your emotional self is essential and requires most of your effort if you are determined to carve out a new and enduring life without opioids.

The Addiction Career

In earlier chapters we looked at the different effects which could be achieved by long-acting and short-acting opioids. You now appreciate that shorter acting opioids are more *reinforcing* because the effect is felt quickly. You also know that the effects wear off quickly too and this is what encourages you to take the opioid multiple times as day. If you are using short acting oral opioids, such as codeine, you may have ended up turning to heroin as, ironically, it is sometimes easier to obtain. From heroin, you are very likely to have progressed from inhaling to injecting, which carries an increased risk of accidental overdose or infection. Your life will have become a round of sourcing, using and recovering from drugs. This is actually a full-time job, and many substance misuse specialists refer to this as a 'career'. Unfortunately, though, this is one of the only careers which offers few rewards – mainly costs. So, until something is done which allows you to have a rest from your career, you will not be able to break the cycle. About 50% of people are able to reduce and detox themselves without professional help. However the evidence suggests that for people who struggle to detox or who have destabilising psychological or social issues in their life, one of the best way to break the cycle and give yourself breathing space to work on your issues, is to replace your short-acting opioids with one that is long-acting, albeit for a short period of time.

Introducing a harm-reduction approach

Let us begin by looking at where many people are when they realise that it is time for them to get some help for their opioid dependence. Most people seek help because of the problems that their drug use is causing them. It is very likely that there are an increasing number of negative consequences which are affecting your everyday life, including physical and mental health, legal and financial as well as social and domestic issues. It is therefore essential to look at a range of goals, both long term and short term, which are aimed at improving health and well-being. These may include:

Short-term goals

- ✓ Reducing any harmful or risky behaviours directly associated with using opioids (for example, using and/or sharing injecting equipment)
- ✓ Reducing any harmful or risky behaviours directly associated with obtaining opioids (for example, buying street drugs, using illegal methods to raise money, such as stealing, sex working, or diversion of family income)
- ✓ Reducing other health issues you may be experiencing by using other substances or medications. For example, you may be drinking excessively or misusing other medications, such as benzodiazepines. If you are using codeine-containing analgesics, you may also be taking excessive amounts of paracetamol or ibuprofen. Excessive or incorrect use of these medicines may cause potentially life-threatening conditions such as liver damage or gastric bleeding

Long-term goals

- ✓ Achieving controlled, non-dependent or non-problematic opioid use
- ✓ Achieving abstinence from opioids
- ✓ Achieving abstinence or controlled use of other substances or medications
- ✓ Building or improving physical and mental wellbeing
- ✓ Building social networks within both the family and community
- ✓ Building resilience in order to protect yourself from relapse

The difficulties experienced in achieving these goals will depend upon the duration and severity of your opioid dependence, and this will also influence the approach to treatment that will suit you best. For people who have only recently started to increase their use of opioids, they may simply be able to reduce by themselves, and, where physical pain is a factor, look to other sources of pain relief. However, where tolerance has developed, and physical and psychological dependence has become established, a longer-term approach, involving experienced healthcare professionals may need to be taken. This approach will start by looking at short term goals, and in particular, reducing harm and risk to yourself and others.

Follow the evidence

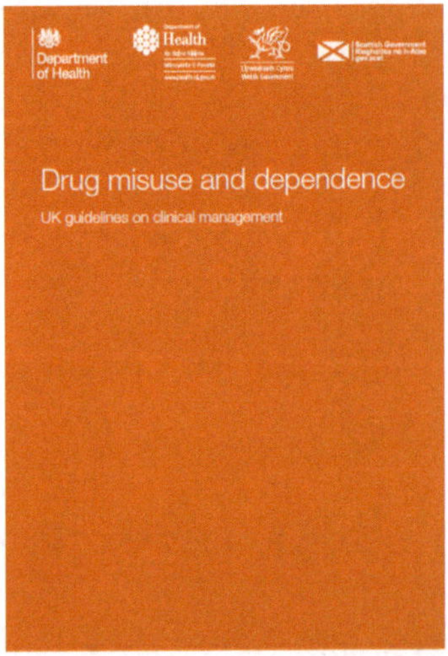

In 2017, the Department of Health commissioned an Independent Expert Working Group, which included treatment service users (patients) and their representatives, to produce a set of evidence-based guidelines entitled *'Drug misuse and dependence: UK guidelines on clinical management'*. These guidelines, also referred to as the *'Orange Guidelines'*, are aimed at healthcare professionals, and are freely available online. They cover both the pharmacological and psychosocial aspects of treating a range of dependencies, including opioid dependence. Whilst these are only guidelines and are not legally binding, they are widely adopted by treatment providers throughout the United Kingdom. This endorsement means that if a treatment provider choses to step outside of this document's recommendation, they will need to justify their actions if things go wrong. Having said that, the general theme throughout these guidelines is that of inclusivity and co-operation. They aim to foster patient and carer engagement, putting patients at the heart of treatment by providing, where possible, appropriate choices dependent on individual need.

Opioid Substitution Treatment (OST)

Opioid Substitution Treatment is viewed as an essential harm-reduction approach to opioid dependence. It means, as the name suggests, replacing the opioid(s) you are taking (you may be using multiple types), with one single, prescribed formulation. To many people, replacing one addictive substance with another seems completely illogical, but there is a sound, evidence-based foundation for doing this which we have already touched upon in previous chapters. Furthermore, the principle that clinicians could legitimately prescribe addictive drugs as part of treatment is not new. In fact, it was set out around a century ago in the Rolleston Report of 1926. This document acknowledged that abstinence should be the long-term goal of everyone who is dependent upon opioids, but that this goal may not be achievable for everyone. For those people where abstinence is not achievable, longer term prescribing should be a legitimate alternative.

The World Health Organisation put both methadone and buprenorphine on their list of essential medicines in 2005. Many countries, mainly those outside of Europe, do not recognise OST as an acceptable treatment option for managing opioid dependence. This may be due to cost as they do not have the internal resources to provide appropriate substance misuse services to match the demand. Alternatively, it is more likely due to cultural factors as in countries like Russia, or Pakistan. Their approach to opioid dependence is sometimes far more punitive, and therefore the only option available to opioid addicted people may be a rapid, non-opioid detoxification, probably with little or no aftercare.

The OST approach to opioid addiction is especially helpful where illicit opioids are being used, and heroin in particular. Most adult drug users in treatment in the United Kingdom still report that heroin is their main problem drug, but there is another large group of people struggling with prescribed or over the counter (OTC) opioids who mainly keep themselves hidden from formal treatment services. Patients using solely prescribed opioids, or OTC opioids such as codeine may, however, be less opioid dependent than those using heroin and may therefore respond to a less intensive treatment. However, to date, there is very little published research into effective approaches for these patients.

For the purpose of clarification, 'published research' means that a formal study has been carried out, and the method used to conduct the study, as well as the findings, have been subjected to peer-review. In other words, the findings have been validated by experts working in that area of medicine, and have then been published in an appropriate journal, for example, The Lancet. Published research does not include an article published in a newspaper, regardless of how credible that newspaper is, or information obtained from a website (for example Wikipedia) or an article identified by using a general internet search engine (as opposed to organisations such as *PubMed* which collates life science journals and articles).

Anyway, regardless of how you arrived in this situation, OST may be an advisable option for you, especially in the short term.

What makes OST effective?

The majority of long acting opioids which are taken orally will last for around 24 hours. If this opioid is prescribed, it means that you will not have to source your own opioids by whatever means you have been adopting. It also means that you will not have to worry about or manage unplanned or uncontrolled withdrawal symptoms, as the long-acting opioid will hold you until your next daily dose.

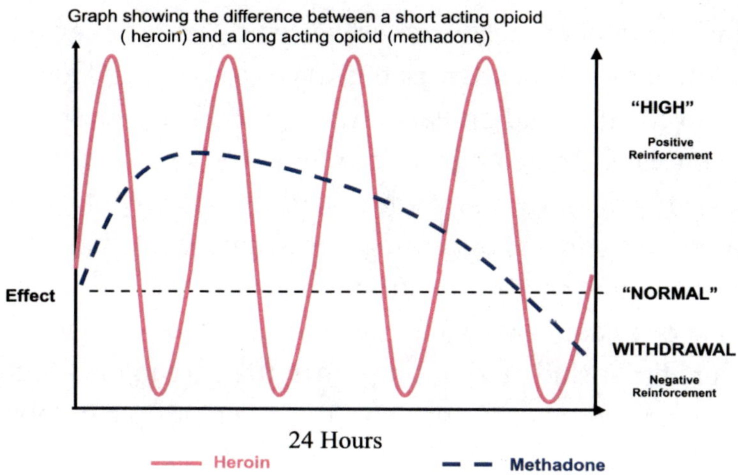

You may, at this point, be wondering why it would not be simpler to just stop taking the opioids and weather the storm of withdrawal; after all, the detox period is a molehill isn't it? About 50% of people are able to detox themselves, but only a proportion of these will be able to remain abstinent. But if you are someone who has tried and failed repeatedly before, bear in mind that going 'cold turkey' is rarely going to be successful unless you get additional support or professional help. Both uncontrolled withdrawal symptoms and a lack of preparation are major causes for relapse. Withdrawal from drugs is not just about stopping them, but preparing sufficiently to be able to climb over the mountain of psychosocial effort. Even if you do manage to become opioid-free, your risk of relapse in the short term is high, especially if you have not built plenty of support around you. In the event that you do go back to opioid use, you also will be exposing yourself to a high risk of overdose, due to the loss of opioid tolerance. It is helpful to view OST as a period of respite which will enable you to build on your resilience and emotional capital. If used properly, it will hold you while you sort out any physical and mental health needs which may have been neglected or caused by your dependence on opioids. The time and headspace this will free up will effectively allow you to start to lift the lid on Pandora's box in a safe, controlled way. It will also enable you to look to the future and plan your life. This may involve dealing with any educational, employment or housing needs as well as addressing any legal problems which may have arisen. Aside from the individual harm-reduction benefits, there is also a huge body of evidence showing that OST also provides wider public health benefits, including reducing crime, the spread of blood-borne infections and overdose by engaging and retaining opioid-dependent people in treatment.

Opioid Substitution Treatment (OST) – When the tail wags the dog

Despite the many obvious harm-reduction benefits to OST, there is, however, a caveat which should be borne in mind before you consider this to be a suitable treatment option for you - after all, no treatment option is a panacea. OST is an excellent tool for helping you get to grips with the chaos in your life. However, whilst the benefits of having a once-daily substitution treatment should now be clear, it will only be effective if you have engaged with psychosocial interventions to support you when you start to lift the lid as you start to reduce or detox. You may, for example, experience a re-emergence distressing thoughts, feelings and memories. On a practical level, you will also need support in adjusting to a new daily routine. For example, sleep may become more of an issue for you as you are likely to be 'awake' for parts of the day when previously you were under the influence or recovering from the effects of opioids. As part of your treatment plan, it is no doubt beneficial to move away from certain environments and people which were associated with your previous opioid use. You will need to fill this new free time constructively with a routine that you have set up for yourself. For some, being on OST may be just plain boring! Ask yourself how you will fill your day and, possibly, your phone book? Write this down as a plan. You don't necessarily need to stick to this plan, but if you are at a loose end, look at the plan and do what it says!

You are also likely to have more disposable income, as you are only paying for your prescription and of course, you will not even be doing this if you are receiving state-funded benefits. This extra money may 'burn a whole in your pocket' begging to be spent on drugs, until you have put it out of reach or spent it. You will need a clear plan as part of your preparation for what you are going to do with your money. It will be very easy to replace the opioids with other substances, especially alcohol. Aside from the fact you may be replacing one addiction with another, drugs such as alcohol will interact with your OST, increasing your risk of developing other health issues, including liver and gut problems and overdose.

Finally, at the risk of being controversial, you may find that your treatment providers are reluctant to plan a treatment exit strategy with you. In previous years, this was certainly the case, because government funding for drug treatment services was based upon targets for engaging and retaining people in treatment, not for helping them to exit. Effectively, the policy makers did not build a 'back door' into their treatment model. This led to a culture of 'learned helplessness' and an aging population of people using pretty high doses of OST into middle-age and beyond. For some people, it has meant remaining on OST for longer than necessary as their drug using 'career' may otherwise have come to a natural end much sooner.

All of these are good reasons for planning your treatment carefully. Take charge and remember, the *Orange Guidelines* support the fact that you should be involved in the decision-making about your treatment as much as possible. It is sensible to view OST as having a beginning, a middle and an end, and make plans for that end by developing an exit strategy, whether it is months or even years away. As we know, life is a journey not an event, and our priorities change as we get older. Remaining too long on OST may mean that you have missed opportunities, or life events, which would have been key motivators for you to move on naturally.

Age of clients in Drug Treatment 2005- 14 *Drug treatment in England 2013-14 (Public Health England)*

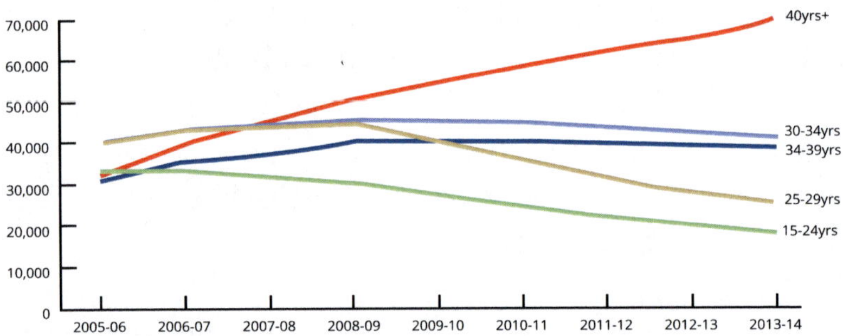

OST- What to expect

Let us now assume that, for reasons you have carefully considered, you feel that OST is the appropriate path for you to take. Being on OST means that an opioid will be prescribed for you, and it is sometimes your general practitioner who will be able to get you started on OST, and sometimes the specialist addiction service. If you want to start OST, your GP is, however, a very good place to start your journey, especially if they have been prescribing opioids for you or you have been buying over-the-counter opioids from pharmacies. GPs will play a key role in your care by managing your other physical health needs, sign posting you to other agencies, and possibly continuing to prescribe your OST for you when things have stabilised.

So, the first thing you must be prepared to be is totally honest. There is no point telling anything but the truth when it comes to your own use of opioids and other substances and, quite honestly, not doing so could put you at risk. Your prescriber (and it may be a nurse or pharmacist, as well as a doctor) will need to ensure that you are, in fact dependent upon opioids. They will want to know the type, quantity and way you are taking them, and to identify any other immediate risks to yourself, such as injecting or sharing needles or any other substances you may be taking, prescribed or otherwise.

At the start of treatment, a key goal for your prescriber will be to provide the most appropriate OST for you, and to prescribe or build up to a dose that will match your existing opioid tolerance so that you feel stable.

Methadone and buprenorphine are the oral opioid agents licensed for use in treating opioid dependence in the United Kingdom and are approved by the National Institute of Health and Clinical Excellence (NICE). They hold the strongest international evidence base of effectiveness in OST. A decision will need to be taken as to which of these two medications would be most appropriate for you. We will look at the differences between methadone and buprenorphine later.

So, in order for your prescriber to determine how much OST to prescribe to prevent both the risk of withdrawals and, more importantly, the risk of overdose, you will need to provide as much accurate information as you can. If you have been using illicit opioids, such as heroin, this will be more difficult to assess but, again, be as accurate as you can about your daily use. In addition to the information you have provided, your treatment provider will also want to carry out additional assessments. These will include assessing your level of dependence. This will involve observing any OWS you may be experiencing, as well as doing drug screening to confirm that you are, indeed, currently taking opioids. The drug screens, most commonly a urine screen, can usually show which type of opioids are in your system. They may also screen for other substances or medications such as benzodiazepines, cannabis, cocaine, amphetamines etc. Do not be concerned about this; you will not be judged. The GP or team will want to see you holistically and will be used to seeing people who use a variety of drugs. They will see OST as a separate intervention but hope that this or their psychosocial interventions will result in you reducing or stopping the other drug use.

It is not necessarily helpful, albeit understandable, to exaggerate your use of opioids and minimise your use of other substances in order to ensure that you are prescribed enough. The GP or treatment team will hopefully be very experienced in recognising your needs and concerns and are there to help and support you, and ultimately keep you safe. They will want to provide you with a safe OST dose, which may not be sufficient to prevent all withdrawal symptoms initially. But if they feel you need it, they will want to build up the dose to a level that you need to prevent all withdrawal symptoms.

Another strategy for keeping you safe is very likely to involve ensuring that your medication is administered to you in a supervised manner. Supervised consumption of OST is a widely used approach and means that you not only obtain your medicine on a daily basis, but you are observed swallowing it or placing it on or under your tongue. This helps to ensure that you do not have any adverse effects from your dose. It also protects you from being pressured into handing over or selling your medication to someone else. Finally, it also protects other people you may be living with, especially children, from the risk of overdose.

Methadone or buprenorphine

There is a very substantial evidence base for the effectiveness of both methadone and buprenorphine, and it is important that you are able to discuss which you think would suit you best with your treatment provider. Both of these medications have distinct pros and cons, and we will look at these in the next chapter. Currently, there remains insufficient evidence to justify recommending one drug over the other and the *Orange Guidelines* state:

"There is no simple formula that can be recommended to determine the suitable clinical choice of methadone or buprenorphine. It is (therefore) essential that clinicians do not exaggerate what is currently known to support one drug over another, so that patients are empowered to make their own decision, taking account of the reasonable informed advice of the prescriber, which also helps the patient to take account of their own personal circumstances."

I would, at this point, like to issue a word of caution. Methadone and buprenorphine are a means to a desired end and not an end in itself – whether harm reduction or abstinence. Although there is an enormous amount of evidence supporting the use of methadone and, indeed buprenorphine, these studies are, in the main, carried out on patients engaged in addiction treatment. This means that the research does not necessarily tell us how people who *did not* chose to engage in treatment services faired. The very nature of addiction means that the people engaged in the research are extremely vulnerable and will be experiencing very high levels of stress. They are therefore more likely to engage in a process that ensures they do not have to manage their addiction alone. The age of opioid dependent individuals in the United Kingdom is increasing, and this may suggest that drugs like methadone are responsible for denying certain people the opportunity of achieving abstinence. Whilst the reduced stigma associated with the use of drugs such as methadone cannot have come soon enough it is, after all, only as affective as the psychosocial support that is provided.

Non-opioid alternatives for detoxification

Throughout this book, I have focused almost entirely on opioids as both the cause and the treatment of opioid dependence. Methadone and buprenorphine as opioid substitution treatments are the go-to options for stabilising patients and, in the majority of cases, helping them to detox. It would be remiss of me not to mention another alternative which may be available for certain people in certain situations. Not everyone wants to use opioid-based medications for withdrawal, especially if their level of dependence is not so high or they need or desire to be opioid-free within a relatively short space of time – I am talking about detoxing over a couple of weeks instead of a few months. Before I say more, you need to understand that there are specific challenges around opting for these medications. These challenges include availability and licensing restrictions.

Alpha$_2$ agonists

Alpha$_2$ agonists have been used for many years in the United Kingdom, and indeed many continents around the world. The fact that they are not opioids offers distinct advantages for certain individuals. Alpha$_2$ agonists include lofexidine and clonidine. Neither of these drugs are Controlled Drugs, and therefore do not cause dependence. They are merely used to manage withdrawal symptoms during the detox process.

Both lofexidine and clonidine are referred to in the *Orange Guidelines*, which states that they:

"are not generally used in detoxification for patients with substantial dependence but may be helpful in relieving symptoms of withdrawal in those who are using small amounts of opioids and are keen to achieve abstinence."

It could be argued that patients with substantial dependence are not likely to be ready for any type of detoxification until the psychosocial aspects of their addiction have been properly managed. When that has happened, these medicines may well then be a useful and appropriate option. Before looking at the potential role of these drugs, let us first look at what is meant by the term Controlled Drug.

What is a Controlled Drug (CD) /medicine?

Strict legal controls are needed for certain medicines which have the potential for causing dependence or for being misused because they may cause serious harm if they are not used correctly. *The Misuse of Drugs Act 1971 (as amended)* divides drugs into 3 classes, A, B and C, with Class A dugs being subject to the tightest restrictions or prohibitions in terms of manufacture, possession and use.

The Misuse of Drugs Regulations 2001 details extra safety measures that must be put in place to make sure they are prescribed, supplied, used and stored safely and legally. CDs include some strong painkillers, such as diamorphine and codeine, some tranquillisers and stimulants, and medicines used to treat dependence, such as buprenorphine and methadone.

The Misuse of Drugs Regulations 2001 divide CDs into five schedules according to their therapeutic usefulness and misuse potential. I have provided more information in the final chapter, '*Legal Stuff*', if you would like to know more about this subject.

Lofexidine and clonidine are not Controlled Drugs, and therefore do not cause dependence. They are merely used to manage withdrawal symptoms during the detox process.

Clonidine
Legal Status: Prescription Only Medicine (not a Controlled Drug)
Licensed for treating hypertension (high blood pressure). Clonidine is not licensed for opioid detoxification.
Brand name in the United Kingdom – Catapres®. (Also known as Kapvay®, and Nexiclon® in other countries)

Clonidine was licensed as an antihypertensive several decades ago. Unfortunately, despite its effectiveness at lowering blood pressure, its side effect profile, in particular sedation, meant that patients didn't like taking it – which is not helpful if you are prescribed it for high blood pressure! However, the lack of product licence did not prevent clonidine from being used to manage OWS throughout the world for many years, due to its effect on noradrenaline.

As a result of this widespread use, there is now extensive evidence of clonidine's effectiveness. Here in the United Kingdom, its side effect profile limits its use mainly to in-patient units. This means that close monitoring of blood pressure and sedation should be carried out during treatment.

Lofexidine
Legal Status: Prescription Only Medicine (not a Controlled Drug)
Licensed for relieving the symptoms in patients undergoing opioid detoxification
Brand name in the United Kingdom – BritLofex®
Brand name in the United States – Lucemyra®

Sadly, supplies of lofexidine in the United Kingdom and Europe ceased in 2018 and, at the time of printing, have not recommenced. It is not known whether lofexidine will be manufactured again in Europe. Lofexidine was licensed for opioid detoxification by the Food and Drink Administration (FDA) in the United States of America and is available under the brand name **Lucemyra**®. Ironically the licence for Lucemyra was granted in the United States in the same year that it was discontinued in Europe. The United Kingdom's loss is therefore the United States' gain as lofexidine is currently the only licensed non-opioid medication in the world.

Lofexidine was originally developed as an alternative anti-hypertensive medication to clonidine with fewer side effects. It did, indeed cause less sedation, but was not effective enough at lowering blood pressure to be licensed for that purpose. As a result, it was abandoned by the pharmaceutical company that had developed it. In 1992, the pharmaceutical company I was employed by, was granted a licence for the use of lofexidine in managing opioid withdrawal symptoms. Lofexidine then became used in a wide range of treatment settings, including the community, in-patient units and prisons until manufacturing ceased in 2018. During the time that lofexidine was available in the United Kingdom, clonidine was rarely used, as clinicians opted for the licensed option. Lofexidine was also easier to manage as it had fewer side effects, which meant that its use was no longer limited to in-patient units. However, now that lofexidine is no longer available, it is likely that clonidine may start to make a come-back. Either way, I think it is important to be aware that there may be medications to help come off opioids that do not involve using opioids. It should be noted that in the United Kingdom, whilst some general practitioners felt comfortable managing patients wishing to detox in this way, the use of $alpha_2$ agonists took place mainly in specialist substance misuse services. This was because the dose level needed increasing rapidly, stabilising and then reducing slowly, as well as blood pressure and pulse monitoring, which meant detoxes were best managed by a prescribing nurse. If this is an option you are considering, you should bear this in mind.

How do lofexidine and clonidine work?

In chapter 5, I explained the relationship between endorphins, opioids and the stress hormone, noradrenaline. You will now understand that when opioids are stopped suddenly, this releases a lot of noradrenaline which, until then, had been supressed by the opioids. This leads to the noradrenaline storm which is responsible for the majority of OWS.

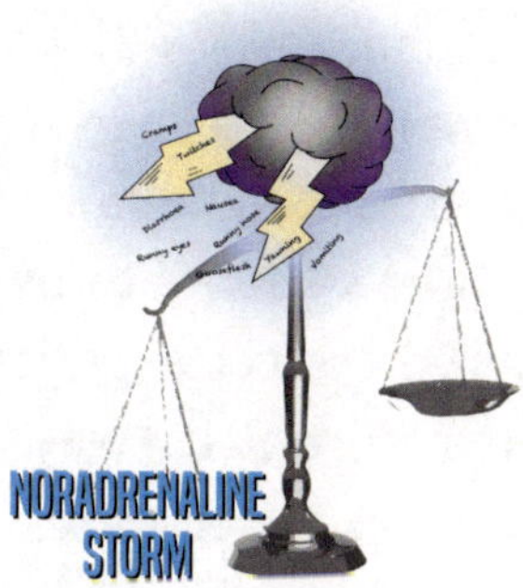

One way to reduce the noradrenaline storm, would be to take opioids again, which would bind to the opioid receptors and push back the noradrenaline. However, there is another way, which does not involve taking more opioids, and this is where the alpha$_2$ agonists come in.

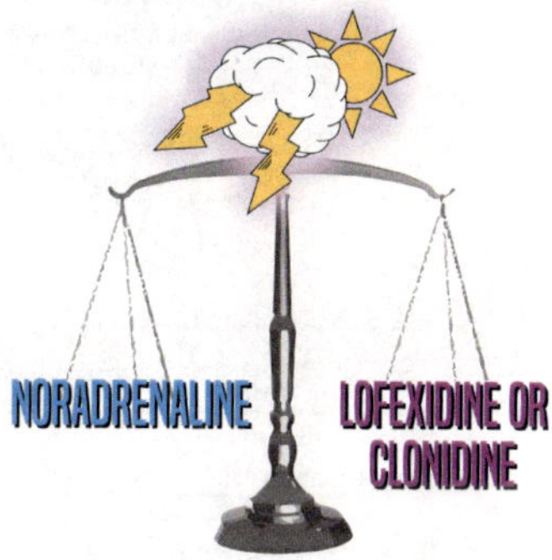

Most of the brain's noradrenaline is produced in a part of the brain called the locus coeruleus (meaning 'little blue spot' in Latin). As opioid tolerance has increased, more alpha$_2$ adrenergic receptors have been produced in association with the increased noradrenaline. Drugs like lofexidine and clonidine work by binding with these receptors and effectively switching off the noradrenaline storm. As the amount of noradrenaline reduces, so do the numbers of alpha$_2$ adrenergic receptors. So effectively, clonidine and lofexidine 'reset' the noradrenaline levels and, as a result, extinguish the noradrenaline storm. This process can take 7 to 10 days when detoxing from short-acting opioids and around 3 weeks for higher dose, longer-acting opioids. The real key to success with alpha$_2$ agonists is to try to match the medication dose with where you are in the withdrawal process. In other words, you need to ensure that you are on the optimum dose of either lofexidine or clonidine on the day you anticipate the peak of withdrawal symptoms to occur. The following chart is based on extensive clinical experience of using lofexidine and demonstrates this in a more visual way.

This chart shows the typical opioid withdrawal pattern depending on the type and dose of opioid you are detoxing from and how lofexidine and clonidine may be used to help to manage the symptoms

Note: In addition to the acute opioid withdrawal lasting 1-2 weeks, you may experience a protracted withdrawal syndrome lasting several weeks or months, especially following high dose or long-term methadone or buprenorphine.

Also be aware that withdrawal from opioids may also unmask symptoms from underlying conditions

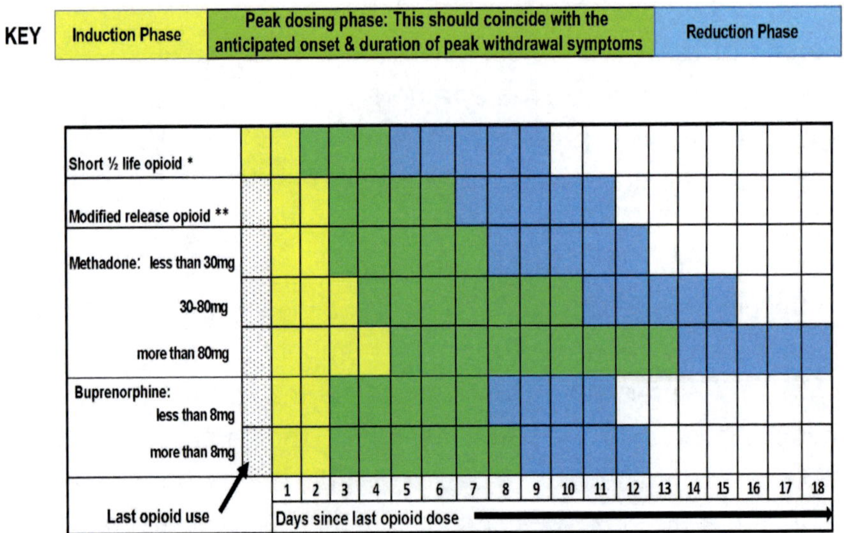

* Examples of short acting opioids Start a2 agonists 6-12 hours after last dose	Heroin, Co-codamol, dihydrocodeine, morphine, tramadol, pethidine
** Examples of modified release opioids Start a2 agonists about 12 hours after last dose, when withdrawal symptoms develop.	MST Continus™, DHC Continus™, Zydol SR™ (Tramadol SR), Temgesic™ (buprenorphine analgesic doses)

With kind permission from Dr Fergus Law

Because $alpha_2$ agonists are not addictive, you should be offered a degree of flexibility around how much you need, and when. This is different from the structured approach to opioid withdrawal that will be put in place if you are trying to reduce gradually through a detoxification process using opioids. It is also likely that you may require additional symptomatic medication to help with particular symptoms, especially sleep. As well as flexible dosing, another advantage of using drugs lofexidine and clonidine to detox means that you can start the relapse prevention medication, naltrexone, quickly. You will find out more about this in the following chapter.

CHAPTER 7
Choosing Your Path

It may have come as a surprise to you to realise how few pharmacological options are available as you embark upon your journey towards recovery and away from opioid dependence. Consider, if you were suffering from depression, or even high blood pressure, your medical team would have a whole armoury of treatment options available to them. However, when it comes to opioid dependence, the mainstay of treatment are drugs which bind directly to the opioid receptors. These consist of just four: methadone or buprenorphine which are used for OST and detoxification, naltrexone, which is used for relapse prevention, and naloxone, which is used for the reversal of overdose. So, before we start to unpick which treatment may suit which person, let us begin with some definitions and terminology.

When we talk about opioid treatments, we use the following terms:

Agonist, partial agonist and antagonist

Agonist and **antagonists** are drugs that act in opposite directions. When an agonist produces an action, an **antagonist** opposes the action. An opioid **agonist** binds with the receptors and makes them produce the same effect as naturally occurring opioids (endorphins). In sufficient doses they can cause an opioid effect, such as euphoria or respiratory depression. An opioid antagonist on the other hand, binds with the receptor but does not activate it. In other words, it causes no opioid effect – no euphoria, no sedation, no respiratory depression, nothing. So, having produce no agonist effect, an antagonist then sits on the receptor, blocking it and preventing agonists from binding to it. The following diagrams should help to explain this a little more clearly.

Full Agonists

It is helpfully to think of your opioid receptors as a lock, and agonists as the keys which fit in the lock and activate the receptors. So, using this analogy, a full agonist fits the lock perfectly and activates it fully.

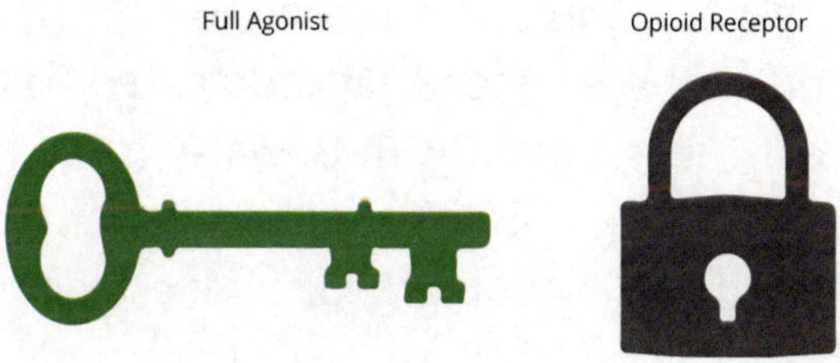

Examples of full agonists include: Morphine, methadone, codeine and heroin

Partial Agonists

A **partial agonist** attaches to the lock but does not fit it perfectly, which means that whilst partial agonists can have similar effects to full agonists, they do not produce them to the same extent as full agonists. They also lose effectiveness at higher doses, which has the advantage that respiratory depression is less likely to happen. Interestingly, when partial agonists are already occupying the lock, other agonists will not be able to fit into the lock at the same time. This again helps to prevent overdose. This blocking effect of partial agonists mean that when heroin or other opioid agonists are used 'on-top' of them, the euphoric effect is reduced or blocked, reducing the positive reinforcement obtained. This in effect reduces the likelihood of further 'on-top' use.

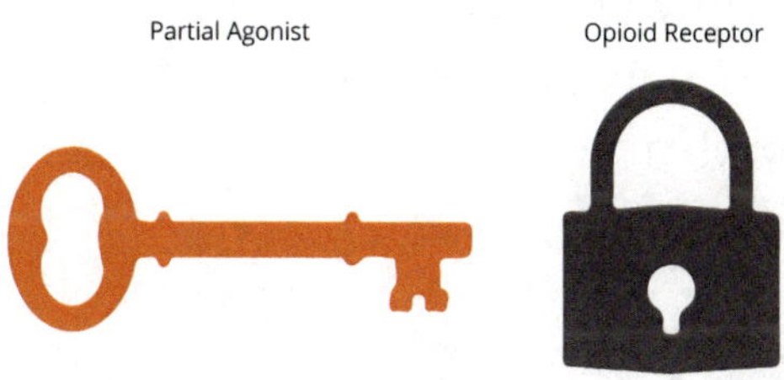

Examples of partial agonists include: Buprenorphine and tramadol

Antagonists

An opioid antagonist attaches itself to the opioid receptor, but instead of activating it, it blocks it and prevents opioids from binding: acting as a kind of blockade, or shield. Furthermore, if the lock is already occupied by a key (full or partial agonist), the antagonist will push the agonist out of the lock and sit there instead. Of course, removing the agonist from the lock will cause opioid withdrawal symptoms. These symptoms will occur very quickly and may continue until the antagonist has worn off and, effectively unblocked the lock. Opioid antagonists play a very useful role in both relapse prevention and the reversal of opioid overdoses.

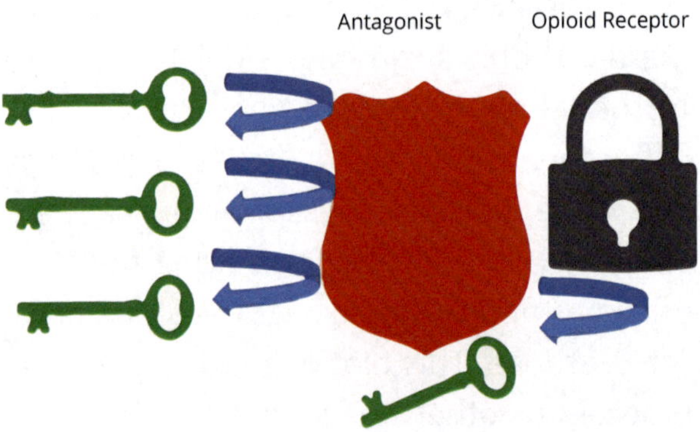

Examples of antagonists include: Naltrexone and naloxone

We will now look more closely at the main medications used in each category. However, instead of beginning with drugs like methadone and buprenorphine, which are used at the start of treatment, I think that it would be helpful to start by describing the drugs which may be used later on in treatment. I hope the reasons for them will soon become clear, so please bear with me.

Naloxone
Legal Status: Prescription Only Medicine
Not a Controlled Drug
Brand name: Prenoxad® (injection) and Nyxoid® (nasal spray)

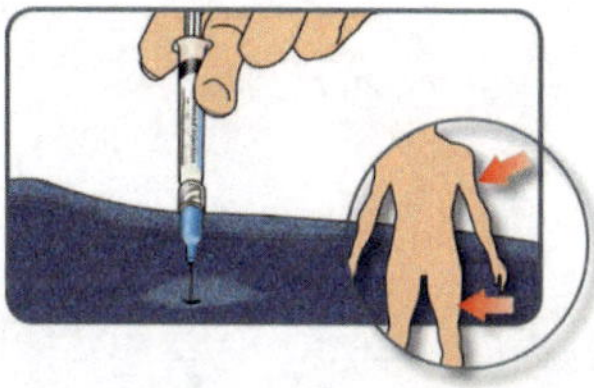

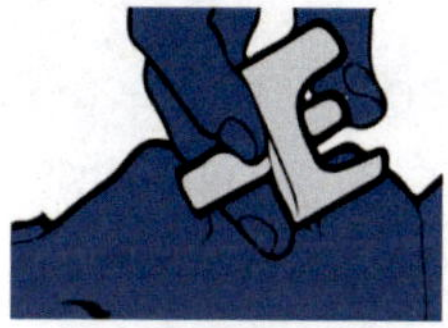

Naloxone is an opioid antagonist which is licensed for the reversal of opioid overdose. It is viewed as a 'rescue therapy' only, which means, as this suggests, that it is used in emergency situations. Naloxone has been shown to save many lives over many years, normally in clinically managed situations (e.g. by a paramedic). These days it is often given directly to drug users regardless of whether they are in the temporary care of a healthcare professional or engaged in formal treatment programme, or regardless of whether they are using prescribed or 'street' opioids'. In other words, the majority of naloxone these days is administered by drug users to drug users, as most opioid overdoses take place in private not clinical settings. In order to allow this to happen, the United Kingdom government put legislation in place to protect individuals who administer a prescription only medicine (POM) that may or may not have been prescribed for them, to the overdose victim to save their life. This is an extremely pragmatic approach, which also helped the medication be used more frequently in situations where it is most needed. Prior to this change in legislation, paramedics were most likely to be the ones administering naloxone to patients in extremely hazardous circumstances. Now, in many cases, the patient has already received naloxone, maybe repeatedly, by the time the emergency services arrive. This has, without doubt, resulted in more lives saved.

Naloxone can be administered in the following ways:

- Injected intramuscularly (IM) - Prenoxad®
- Nasal spray - Nyxoid®
- injected intravenously (IV)
- Injected via intravenous infusion (used in a hospital setting)

When naloxone is administered, it attempts to bind with the opioid receptors and prevent any opioids from attaching. If opioids are already present, it will actually remove them from the receptors and bind there instead. If the receptors were flooded with opioids to the point that respiratory depression had occurred, this process would be reversed, and the patient would recover. However, by removing the opioids from your receptors, you will go into immediate withdrawal, experiencing all of the unpleasant symptoms we have already discussed. It is just as if the naloxone is carrying out an extremely rapid, unplanned and deeply uncomfortable, detoxification. This is considered a small price to pay for saving a life, although not all recipients of naloxone necessarily agree! There have been reports of the person administering the naloxone being assaulted by the overdose victim, who is oblivious to how close a call it was and is only angry about the lost 'hit' and the urgent need to find more drugs in order to stave off the withdrawal symptoms.

Naloxone cannot be delivered in an oral formulation, for two extremely valid reasons. Firstly, naloxone is extensively metabolised by the liver and it would therefore require huge doses (maybe 50 times greater) in order to have the beneficial effect. Therefore, a route into the body that avoids that process is essential. Secondly, it would not be possible for someone who has overdosed to swallow a tablet, as they will very likely be drowsy, unconscious or in respiratory arrest. An injection of naloxone starts to work within minutes, which is fast enough to bring someone round from an overdose in most situations. However, as we already know, what goes up quickly, comes down quickly, and the effects of the naloxone will wear off after 30 to 90 minutes. This short duration of action could therefore result in the patient 'going over' (overdosing) again if long-acting opioids have been taken, because the effects of the naloxone will wear off quickly, and any residual opioids will re-attach themselves to the now-vacant receptors. It is therefore recommended to call an ambulance after naloxone has been given. If someone has not responded within 2-3 minutes of the first dose of naloxone, then naloxone should be administered again, and possibly multiple times in order to ensure a positive outcome. Of course, where a patient is in hospital, the naloxone can be administered for as long as is required via an IV infusion.

Naltrexone
Legal Status: Prescription Only Medicine
Not a Controlled Drug
Brand name (Opioid/alcohol dependence): Adepend®
Maintenance dose 50mg/day (or higher doses 3 times a week)

Naltrexone is also an opioid antagonist, but unlike naloxone, it is licensed to maintain abstinence in people previously dependent upon opioids. Naltrexone is also licensed to maintain abstinence in people who have been dependent upon alcohol too, but that will not be covered here. As an antagonist, naltrexone shares many of the properties of its sister, naloxone, but it is much longer acting. It too, will remove opioids from the receptor sites and precipitate opioid withdrawal in the process. Like naloxone, it will then occupy the receptors, preventing any further opioid effect until the naltrexone has worn off. This is how it can act as an effective relapse prevention agent. It will not stop you trying to use, but by reducing cravings and blocking the effects of opioids, naltrexone will provide a kind of shield or safety net which will allow you breathing space. It you do use opioids impulsively whist taking naltrexone, the breathing space allows you to decide whether you want to remain abstinent and continue to use the naltrexone or to stop the naltrexone and return to the opioids. This breathing space can effectively help to prevent a lapse turning into a relapse. Longer acting formulations, like the depots and the implants, have the advantage that you don't have to worry about taking a tablet regularly, and they provide a smooth blood level which reduces anxiety and craving, and a much higher percentage of people remain abstinent. Research has shown that longer acting depot naltrexone is effective for the person and cost effective. It is thought that the even longer-acting implants will be more advantageous for people wanting to maintain abstinence.

Naltrexone is available in the following formulations

- Oral tablet (50mg)
- Depot – this lasts one month. It is not currently licensed in the United Kingdom but may be available through some private clinics. The depot is licensed in the United States (Vivitrol®) for both opioid and alcohol addiction
- Implant – these can last for up to 9 months but are not currently licensed anywhere in the world. They may also be

> available through some private clinics in the United Kingdom. If you plan to go abroad to have an implant, take care that the clinic is using an implant that complies with the GMP (good manufacturing practice), which are the required manufacturing standards. You can find out more about the use of unlicensed medicines in 'Legal Stuff'.

So, you will note that whilst naltrexone has the same pharmacological effect as naloxone, it is used in a different way. Naltrexone tablets are taken once daily (they can also be taken in higher doses 3 times a week) which means that they are able to block the receptors for 24 hours, as opposed to the 30-90 minutes seen with naloxone. Naltrexone is not addictive, does not result in tolerance and yet is probably the most under-used treatment option for opioid dependence. It absolutely does what it says on the tin - it prevents any opioid effect for as long as you take the tablets - and therein lies most of the problem. For a multitude of reasons, some real, some false, very few people request it. Very few of those who request it, are able to start it and, if they do start it, very few remain on it for more than a few weeks. It is easy to see why people are more likely to engage in a treatment which offers them the positive reinforcement of an opioid (as with OST), rather than a drug like naltrexone which offers no immediate positive reinforcement. However, there are so few treatment choices that if there is a medication that protects you from relapse, why wouldn't you at least give it some consideration? I will try to dissect this issue and, hopefully, give naltrexone a fair hearing at the very least.

Common barriers to naltrexone

In the previous chapter, I alluded to the absence of a back door in drug treatment services. By this I mean that once within a treatment service, it is hard to leave as there are relatively few systems in place to help people achieve sustained abstinence. Services have traditionally focussed on opioid maintenance and harm reduction, rather than supporting abstinence. It therefore stands to reason that if most people seeking treatment are being held on OST, very few of them will achieve a planned abstinence and, those that do, are unlikely to be offered naltrexone for a number of reasons. These included the following:

Funding: Naltrexone used to be considered to be an expensive treatment and, back in the early 1990s, when only methadone was available, it probably was by comparison. This argument no longer stands up, given the flurry of newer, more costly products, including the range of buprenorphine formulations now available. Furthermore, naltrexone was viewed by general practitioners as a specialist product and one which had to be initiated in a specialist setting. In fact, the original product licence actually stated this. As a result, many GPs did not feel comfortable initiating it. There was also concern about maintaining someone on naltrexone, despite the fact that many GPs were maintaining people on OST. The likely reason for this stems from concerns about loss of tolerance and the risk of overdose in the event that the individual suddenly stopped taking naltrexone and started using opioids again. In this scenario, it is unlikely that someone would inform their treatment team that they wished to stop the naltrexone and start using opioids again and would therefore be unsupported.

Initiation: This probably accounts for one of the biggest barriers to naltrexone being used.

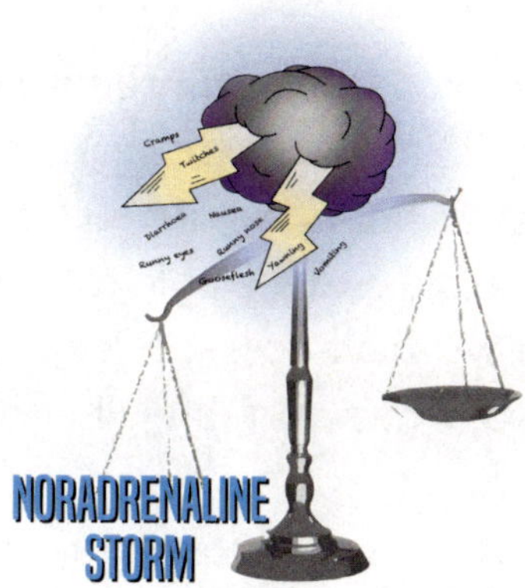

As you now know, if you take an opioid antagonist (naltrexone) at the same time as an opioid agonist (methadone), the antagonist will push the agonist off the receptor and cause withdrawal symptoms. Remember that while you have been using opioids, they have been keeping all of that noradrenaline at bay. So, when naltrexone pushes the methadone off the receptor, you will experience a surge of noradrenaline – the 'noradrenaline storm', together with all of the unpleasant symptoms that go with it.

Whilst getting the opioids out of your system is essential for saving someone from a fatal overdose, as we saw in the naloxone section, this is not appropriate for someone who has not taken an overdose. Imagine that you have been working hard to reduce your opioid use for weeks, or even months. You have just completed the final detoxification and are planning to start naltrexone treatment as part of your relapse - prevention programme. Even though you have taken your last dose of methadone (or buprenorphine), it will remain in your system for 7- 10 days, maybe longer for methadone or 3-4 days for buprenorphine. If you take naltrexone too soon, the naltrexone will push the remaining methadone off the receptors, causing withdrawal symptoms. The end of a detoxification is an extremely vulnerable time, so experiencing unexpected and unpleasant symptoms at this stage could lead to a full-blown relapse. This clearly means that to prevent withdrawal symptoms you must be completely free of opioids before you can start taking naltrexone.

Naltrexone, like buprenorphine and methadone, is a long-lasting drug. Once it is sitting on your receptors, it will remain there for at least 24 hours. So, if you have withdrawal symptoms on naltrexone, no opioids will be able to break through this blockade, meaning that you will have to experience the 'noradrenaline storm' until the naltrexone has worn off, albeit supported by symptomatic medications.

In order to address the risk of causing prolonged withdrawal symptoms, the original product licence for naltrexone stated that, prior to initiation, an injection of naloxone (known as a naloxone challenge test) should be given to test the patient, to see if they were free from opioids. Remember that naloxone lasts for minutes, not hours, so if it did cause withdrawal symptoms, they won't have lasted very long. Regardless of this, imagine the anxiety of sitting in a clinic, waiting to be given an injection of naloxone, knowing there was every likelihood it was going to make you feel very ill! Hopefully it is now easy to see why, a) it was recommended that initiation should take place in a specialist setting and b) why uptake was so poor!

However, things have moved on a lot from there. The newer licence now says that a naloxone challenge test is no longer required if it can be verified that the patient is opioid-free. Verification can easily be done using a urine screen or other drug screen. Furthermore, the introduction of buprenorphine means that the required gap between opioid and naltrexone can be far shorter – only 3 to 4 days. Buprenorphine itself, can also precipitate withdrawal in people already taking opioids, and as a result, treatment providers are now far more experienced at transferring individuals from one medication to another and back again. We will look more closely at buprenorphine later in this chapter.

Psychological impact and urban myths: If you have spent months, years or decades using substances you will be used to taking a drug and expecting some kind of response. In addition, when abstinent you will be trying to learn or relearn coping strategies for your new opioid-free life; you may feel unusually clear headed (which may not have been the case for years or decades), and this can be frightening and stressful.

With naltrexone, you take it and nothing tangible happens – absolutely nothing, so you may feel that you are being cheated by the lack of drug effect. Taking a tablet that doesn't make you feel *anything* is a completely alien concept, especially if your automatic response to managing stress has been to use opioids. It will take a fair amount of work to reprogramme this response, there is no quick fix. Alternatively, you may also wish to test the naltrexone to see if the blockade works. About 50% of people who take naltrexone will, at some point, try to use opioids at the same time either to see if it is working or as an automatic response to a trigger to use opioids. Once again, if you challenge the blockade and take opioids on top of naltrexone, you will not get an effect from the opioid.

One of the very common myths that exists around naltrexone is that if you take opioids whilst taking naltrexone, it makes you very unwell. This is simply not true. I believe that this relates to confusing naltrexone with disulfiram (Antabuse®), which is the medication offered to alcoholics to help them maintain abstinence. If they drink alcohol on top of disulfiram, they will indeed become very ill. On very rare occasions, patients *have* been able to over-ride the naltrexone blockade, but this has required repeated use, at high doses. To attempt this is extremely dangerous and can result in an overdose situation.

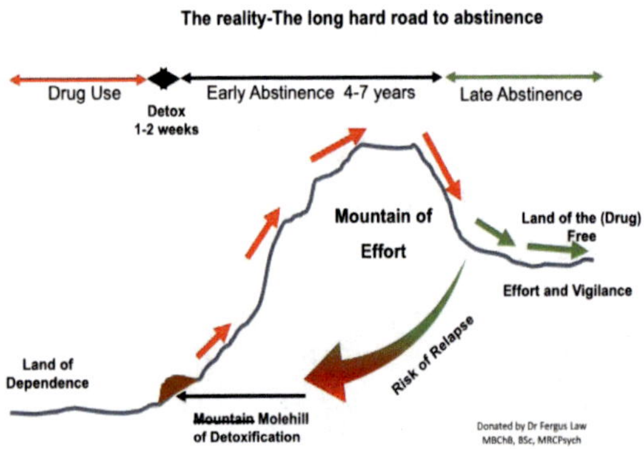

Psychosocial support: No treatment for dependence is a cure, and naltrexone is no different. It is simply a crutch to help you along the road for a period of time until you are able to walk without it – until you are coping well with the challenges of being abstinent and have built up your coping strategies. Having strategies in place to support you at every stage of the journey is essential, especially when you are opioid free. For a lot of people, moving away from their old using networks is extremely beneficial. Some people will benefit from additional support in a residential setting, especially if you have struggled to remain abstinent in the community. Many residential rehabs have a '12 step' approach to treatment which is based upon the principles of the Alcoholics Anonymous fellowship and demands abstinence from all psychoactive substances. There is an ongoing debate as to whether taking naltrexone should be permitted in some of these centres, where the aim is to help you to manage life without any pharmaceutical help. Other centres take a different approach and see naltrexone as a crutch which provides additional support early on at what is a very vulnerable stage in recovery.

Side effects: Some people report stomach complaints such as abdominal pain, nausea and vomiting, diarrhoea and constipation. Most side-effects resolve within 2 weeks of starting naltrexone, as they are related to the body getting used to the drug being present. However, as some of the remaining symptoms are also part of the protracted OWS, it may well be that this is what the people who experienced these symptoms were reporting. Headaches are fairly common at the start of treatment, as are sleep disorders and anxiety, but again, these can also be part of the underlying conditions that lead to the use of opioids in the first place. If the headaches do not go away, it may be related to the naltrexone. With side-effects that are related to the drug and which do not go away, you have to weigh up whether the benefits of continuing the drug outweigh the drawbacks of the side-effects. Many people decide that putting up with a headache for a few months is worth it to ensure that they do not relapse.

Naltrexone has been used for a wide range of addictions, including gambling, alcohol and food. It has been used to treat obese patients at huge doses (6 times the recommended dose) and as a result, changes in some patients' liver blood tests were identified. As a result, liver function tests should be taken at the start and during treatment. Interestingly, naltrexone, in combination with the antidepressant bupropion, is now licensed in the United Kingdom for the treatment of obesity under the brand name Mysimba®. The quantity of naltrexone in Mysimba is 8mg, as opposed to the 50mg used to treat alcohol and opioid dependence.

Pain Management: Because naltrexone blocks the effects of opioids, it will mean in the event that pain relief is required, opioids will not work. It is advisable to carry an alert card, such as the one below, in case of serious emergency situations so that the treatment team caring for you can manage your pain in a different way. As you are recovering from opioid dependence though, it is in any case, probably advisable to avoid opioids and choose different ways to manage any pain.

TO MEDICAL PERSONNEL TREATING ME IN AN EMERGENCY FOR PAIN	Name & phone no. of the prescriber or clinic who prescribed the NALTREXONE
This patient is taking the oral opioid antagonist naltrexone hydrochloride (Adepend®) If this patient should require analgesia and a non-opioid agent is adequate, it should be used. If analgesia with an opioid becomes necessary, the amount of opioid required to achieve a given level of analgesia may be greater than usual and the resulting respiratory depression may be deeper and more prolonged. A rapidly acting analgesic with a short half to minimise the period of respiratory depression is preferred. The amount of analgesic administered should be titrated to the needs of the patient. The patient should be monitored closely by appropriately trained personnel in a hospital setting.	Name of Prescriber: .... Phone No. of Clinic: .... Pharmacy & Phone No: .... Name of Patient: .... Patient's Phone No: .... Date of Issue: ..../........./............

Ending treatment with naltrexone: Assuming you have no serious side-effects, you can remain on naltrexone for as long as you need it. This can mean weeks, months or years. Naltrexone does not cause tolerance, so you can just stop taking it without fear of any withdrawal effects. However, because you have been abstinent form opioids, your tolerance to the effects of opioids will have dropped completely.

You will, effectively, be opioid-naïve once again. This means that if you start to use the same amount of opioids you were taking previously, you will be at serious risk of an overdose, especially in the first month of being abstinent. This is one of the key concerns that treatment providers have regarding naltrexone, and the main reason that prescribers are happier to prescribe OST. Their priority is to keep you safe, and the early months, especially following detoxification, are extremely vulnerable times in terms of relapse.

Buprenorphine
Legal Status: Prescription Only Medicine
Class C; Schedule 3 Controlled Drug/Medicine (CD)
Average daily dose is between 12 and 16mg
Maximum recommended dose 32mg/day
The product licence for buprenorphine states that you should be on the equivalent of 30mg or less of methadone before switching to buprenorphine. However, extensive clinical experience over more than two decades has proven that it is possible to switch safely to buprenorphine from doses of 60-80mg of methadone.
Brand Names (all formulations licensed for opioid dependence): Buvidal®, Espranor®, Prefibin®, Subutex®, Suboxone®

Buprenorphine is licensed for the management of opioid dependence. It is broken down extensively by the liver and therefore cannot be given as an oral tablet. Instead, it is currently available in the following formulations:

- Sublingual tablets (buprenorphine only): 0.4mg, 2mg, 8mg. (Brand name Prefibin® Subutex®)
- Sublingual tablets plus naloxone (ratio 4:1): 2mg, 8mg. (Brand name Suboxone®)
- Oral lyophilisate wafer – a type of tablet that dissolves on the

tongue more rapidly than the sublingual tablets. Buprenorphine only: 2mg, 8mg. (Brand name Espranor®)

- Oral film – -a film that you can stick to the inside of your cheek for it to dissolve, which has the advantage that once stuck, cannot be removed. Also contains naloxone (not currently licensed in UK)
- Prolonged-release solution for injection weekly or monthly (buprenorphine only). Various doses (Brand name Buvidal®)

You may be aware that buprenorphine transdermal patches are also available under a range of brand names e.g. Bunov®, Bupeaze®, Buplast®, Bupramyl®, Butec®, BuTrans®,Carlosafine®, Hapoctasin®, Panitaz®, Reletrans®, Relevtec®, Sevodyne®, Transtec®, Whist patches are occasionally used to treat opioid dependence, they are most commonly used for pain management. Injectable preparations and sublingual tablets (e.g Temgesic® and Tephine®) are also available for managing pain, but the dosage required is rarely high enough to treat addiction. For example, the maximum dose for Temgesic® is 400 *micrograms* every 8 hours, whereas the maximum recommended daily dose for buprenorphine for Subutex® is 32 *milligrams* (i.e. 10 times the maximum daily dose used for pain).

What are the advantages of buprenorphine?

So, what makes buprenorphine an appropriate medication for the treatment of opioid dependence? Buprenorphine is a partial agonist which binds tightly to the opioid receptors (it is often referred to as a 'sticky' drug) but does not stimulate them as much as a full agonist, such as heroin, codeine or methadone does. As a result, buprenorphine produces less 'euphoria' and leaves you clearer headed or feeling more 'normal'. This theoretically means that buprenorphine is less likely to lead to addiction (although physical dependence can occur), and this is reflected in its schedule 3 CD status (whereas methadone is schedule 2). Buprenorphine is a particularly interesting drug because, as well as having agonist properties, it also has antagonist properties. As you now know, antagonists are able to remove opioids that are already bound to the opioid receptors, precipitating opioid withdrawal symptoms. Once the antagonists are sitting on the receptors, they then provide a shield, or blockade, preventing more opioids from attaching to the receptors, especially at buprenorphine doses of 16mg per day or more. This means that buprenorphine is not only able to deliver a milder opioid effect than methadone, but it also prevents or reduces the effects of other opioids that may then be used 'on top' of the buprenorphine. Remember, the effects of too much opioid not only lead to euphoria, but also potentially fatal respiratory depression. Buprenorphine has, what is commonly referred to as, a 'ceiling effect' on its ability to depress our breathing or respiration. In other words, once the receptors are flooded with buprenorphine, the drug can just sit there without causing respiratory depression.

Thus, buprenorphine provides protection from opioid overdose, making it a safer option than full agonists like methadone. Its long duration of action, especially at doses of 16mg daily and above also means that it can be taken every other day if required.

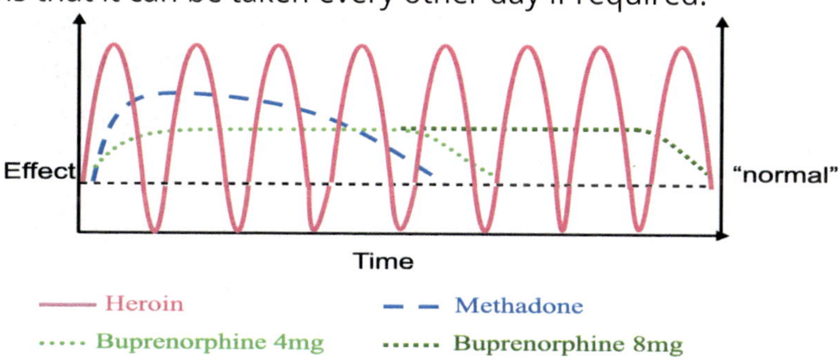

However, it is important to note here that whilst buprenorphine antagonist properties do indeed provide protection, it would be dangerous to give the impression that it is not possible to go into respiratory depression whilst taking buprenorphine. Overdoses have occurred, especially when buprenorphine has been used with other drugs which can also cause respiratory depression, such as benzodiazepines and alcohol.

Buprenorphine as a detox medication

Another advantage of buprenorphine has as a 'sticky drug' is that it comes away (dissociates) from the receptors very slowly. This means that any withdrawal effects are milder than are experienced with full agonists, and any additional support required from symptomatic medications may be minimal.

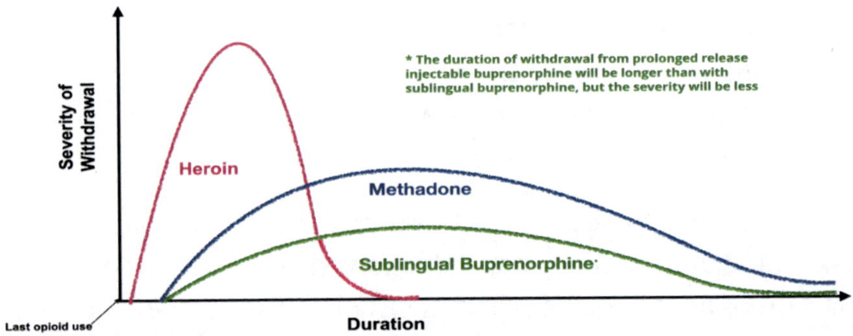

The *Orange Guidelines* state that '*Buprenorphine doses can be reduced initially by 2mg every two weeks or so, with final reductions being around 400 micrograms. Patients report being able to reduce buprenorphine doses more quickly than methadone*'.

I suspect at this stage you may be thinking that buprenorphine pretty much ticks all of the boxes when it comes to OST and, indeed detoxification. Well for the right person, it certainly does offer a lot of benefits over a full agonist such as methadone:

- It is a schedule 3 CD which means there will be fewer restrictions on prescribing and dispensing
- It has opioid agonist properties- albeit milder
- It is safer in overdose
- It can be taken every other day (or weekly or monthly by injection)
- It is easier to detox from than methadone
- Towards the end of a methadone detox, you can switch to buprenorphine to finish off the detox
- It also acts a bit like naltrexone and blocks the euphoria from 'on top' use of other opioids, and the higher the dose the better it blocks

What are the disadvantages of buprenorphine?

The partial agonist effect- feeling normal: Buprenorphine is able to bind to all of the opioid receptors, but it does not fit the lock as well as a full agonist. This means that you do not get the full opioid effect. Whilst this may be ideal if your dependence is fairly mild and of short duration, it may not suit everybody, especially if you have been using opioids to self-medicate for severe emotional pain. According to the product licence, buprenorphine should be used as a 'substitution treatment for opioid drug dependence, within a framework of medical, social and psychological treatment'. If you are keeping your emotions at bay with opioids like heroin or methadone, by taking buprenorphine, you will be partially 'lifting the lid' and need to be prepared for that.

The antagonist effect- precipitated withdrawal: As you now know, opioid antagonists will displace opioids that are already in your body, precipitating opioid withdrawal. In order to minimise this, you will need to wait at least 12 hours after you last took a short-acting opioid, or 24 to 36 hours after taking a long acting opioid before taking your first dose of buprenorphine. In short, starting treatment with buprenorphine may mean that you will have to undergo some level of discomfort first. This is not insurmountable, as there are non-opioid medications which are available to support you (we covered OWS management in the previous chapter). Treatment providers should also be extremely used to initiating patients onto buprenorphine and will have well-established protocols in place to guide you.

The antagonist effect- blocking the euphoria from on top use: As mentioned previously, buprenorphine can act like a shield and protect you from the euphoric effects of 'on top' opioid use. If, during your initial assessment, you have underestimated your daily use, you may experience withdrawal symptoms. If these symptoms are due to an inadequate buprenorphine dose, you may not be able to manage these by 'topping up' with other opioids. Instead, you will need to inform your prescriber and request a dose increase. There should not be an issue with increasing the dose, as the goal of OST is to stabilise you and reduce the harm you have been doing. Prescribing a sub-standard dose of any opioid will not achieve this goal.

Some prescribers may offer you a choice as to whether you would like a higher blocking dose of buprenorphine to prevent on-top use or a lower dose just sufficient to prevent withdrawal symptoms. The logic of this is that although the lower dose will have some blocking effect, if you are not yet ready to stop on-top use completely, you may still get some benefit from on-top use. The potential advantage of this approach, is that it may reduce the number of dropouts from buprenorphine treatment, allowing you time to gradually adapt to being on the drug and adapting to a new routine.

Potential for misuse: I said at the start of this section that the profile of buprenorphine means that it is potentially safer and less addictive than full agonists. That is true if buprenorphine is being used in the manner intended, i.e. as prescribed. The sublingual tablets in particular, are open to misuse and all of the associated harms, as the tablets can be crushed and the powder then either snorted or injected. The prolonged-release solution Buvidal is relatively new in the United Kingdom, with the first licence being granted in 2018, and is not open to this type of misuse. Likewise, the wafer, Espranor, dissolves so quickly on the tongue that diversion is almost impossible.

Buprenorphine has also proved extremely problematic in custodial settings. Whilst a large number of buprenorphine prescriptions are issued to patients in the community who are able to take their medication at home without supervision is a requirement in a secure environment.

During my pharmaceutical career, I visited numerous prison-based substance misuse services and heard and saw this issue first-hand. Virtually no medication, and certainly not a CD, are supplied for the prisoners to have in their possession. Instead, they would be closely supervised to ensure that the medication was taken by the correct patient and not secreted by them in order to sell or give to a third party or to accumulate for their own use at a later time. I would frequently meet staff who had reported that either they or a colleague had been assaulted by prisoners trying to obtain buprenorphine from the clinics, or about prisoners being bullied for their medication. Furthermore, because buprenorphine came in tablet form, it was easier to smuggle in and hide within the prison than, say, heroin or methadone liquid. Once the tablets arrived inside the prison walls they would be sold for huge profit. It was not uncommon to hear anecdotes which claimed that a single 8mg 'Subbie' (Subutex) tablet had a value on the wings of between £40 and £60 - 4-6 times its street value outside of prison. The knock-on effect of this was huge debts being run up inside, which would spill out into the community, resulting in families and friends being expected to cover these debts. Here in the United Kingdom, methadone remains the most widely used opioid treatment in secure environments at present because it is most likely to be taken by the person it is intended for. The rapidly dissolving wafer of buprenorphine (Espranor) is superior to the sublingual buprenorphine tablets in reducing diversion in the prison environment, and it is anticipated that the prolonged-release buprenorphine injection (Buvidal) could also resolve this issue.

In order to try to overcome the potential for misuse of buprenorphine tablets, the manufacturers of the original sublingual tablet launched a new formulation onto the market. This formulation was a sublingual tablet of buprenorphine which also contained naloxone. The first buprenorphine/naloxone combination available in the United Kingdom was called Suboxone and that was launched in 2006, some eight years after the launch of its sister product, Subutex. The rationale behind this combination was as follows; when the combination tablet is taken sublingually as intended, the buprenorphine will have the desired effect but the naloxone (the short-acting, fast-working opioid antagonist), when taken sublingually, does not interfere with the buprenorphine as so little naloxone is absorbed from the mouth and gut. However, if the combination is injected, the naloxone will become active and precipitate withdrawal. In effect, instead of acting as an overdose 'rescue therapy' the naloxone was being used as an 'aversion therapy' designed to discourage further injecting.

It is a principle of good practice not to give medication to a patient that doesn't need it, and which may cause harm. Medication should only be given to the group of patients in whom its benefit is likely to outweigh its risks. If there was a test which could reliability indicate who would use or allow others to use their medication in an unauthorised way, then the naloxone would only be added to the buprenorphine for those patients. However, no such reliable test is available, and therefore naloxone (which is thought to be relatively low in harm) is given to both those who may benefit from it and those who won't.

Espranor® Oral lyophilisate

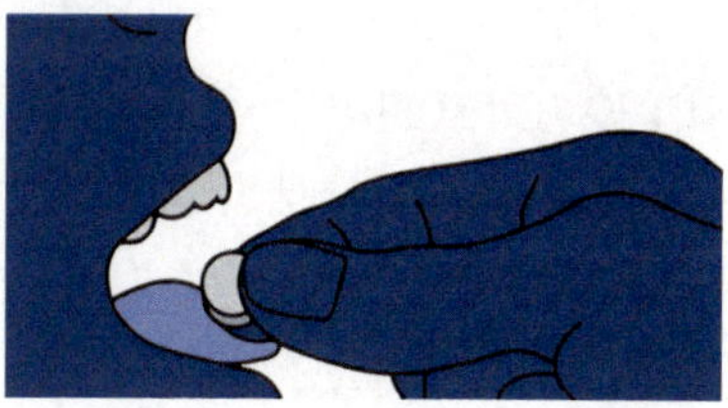

Espranor is different from sublingual buprenorphine tablets. Espranor should be placed *on* the tongue and is absorbed into the bloodstream through the tongue's surface very quickly – usually in less than 15 seconds. This is very different from sublingual buprenorphine tablets which are placed under the tongue. The product licence for sublingual tablets states that the time taken to dissolve is between 5 and 10 minutes. This rapid absorption means that diversion is much more difficult with Espranor and is the main reason that it is used in secure environments.

It is important to note that, because of the different way the drug is absorbed into the body, you will need a lower dose of Espranor than with the sublingual tablets. As you know, there are lots of factors that can affect how much of a drug actually gets you're your system, for example, 100% of drug that is injected into a vein gets into your system, whereas as little as 5% of a drug that is swallowed may get in to your system because it can be affected the liver, other medicines you have taken, as well as food you have consumed. The way Espranor gets into your system is different from the way Subutex or Suboxone gets into your system. Studies have shown that as much as 30% more buprenorphine gets into your system with Espranor than with an equivalent sublingual tablet. As a result, the daily dose will be lower with Espranor. It also means that you cannot necessarily swap at the same dose between the two formulations, wafer and sub-lingual tablet, as this could increase the risk of overdose.

Espranor was launched on to the market in 2017, around the time that the *Orange Guidelines* were published. As a result, the guidelines could not include any guidelines in the document. However, they did state that rapid-dispersal forms of buprenorphine (such as Espranor) may be of clinical benefit by enabling simpler supervised consumption.

Buvidal® Prolonged-release solution for injection

The availability of long-acting injections which can provide cover for one week or one month, has the potential for removing the need for supervised consumption of opioid medication due to concerns about its misuse. Buvidal was granted a licence for use in the United Kingdom in 2018. This means that it also does not appear in the

Orange Guidelines. However, in 2019, the National Institute for Health and Care Excellence (NICE) approved the use of Buvidal and published guidance about it which stated:

'Buprenorphine prolonged-release injection may be an option where there is a risk of diversion of opioid substitution medicines or concerns about the safety of medicines stored at home. It may also be an option for people who have difficulties adhering to daily supervised opioid substitution medication, such as for people who are working or in education.

Buprenorphine prolonged-release injection may have a place in treating opioid dependence in people in custodial settings, where the risk of diversion and time needed for supervised consumption currently leads to challenges in supplying supervised medicines safely.'

This pretty much covers most people living with opioid dependence! Buvidal can be given as a weekly or monthly injection. The benefits of this will be clear to both patients and treatment services. There are many thousands of opioid-dependent people trying to live relatively normal lives, caring for families or holding down a job. Regular visits to a pharmacy create many challenges for these people, especially for daily supervised consumption of medication. A weekly or monthly depot injection also removes the additional risks around accidental or deliberate overdose which occur as a result of 'take home' doses of oral OSTs. A long-acting injection also protects both staff and patients from being victims of actual or threatened violence in a prison setting. Security issues in prisons will often influence the treatment options that are available to you and an alternative treatment option to methadone is likely to be welcomed by prisoners and staff alike.

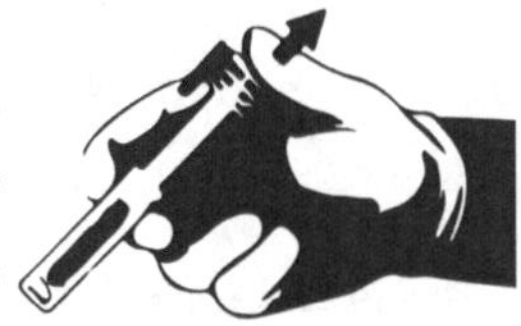

The manufacturers of Buvidal pre-filled syringes use a patented technology, FluidCrystal®, to deliver a depot injection of buprenorphine under the skin. This technology drug means that the buprenorphine is slowly released over a week or a month.

As well as the convenience of a weekly or monthly dosing schedule, blood levels will be maintained even more smoothly, without the peaks and troughs in drug effect that occur with oral medications. The extended duration of action means that the withdrawal, whilst longer lasting than with its sublingual cousin, is likely to be even more gentle.

There is a wide range of syringe strengths available, which means that there is flexibility around dosing with Buvidal. Calculating the equivalent dose of Buvidal compared to the oral formulations is simple. A dose of 16mg a day sublingual tablets is equivalent to 24mg weekly Buvidal and 96mg monthly Buvidal. This is because Buvidal is a subcutaneous injection and is therefore not broken down by the liver. As a result, less is needed to deliver the same effect. There is potential for people who want to change from a daily tablet to a weekly or monthly injection to feel anxious that they will not be covered, or to feel 'short-changed', so it is important that this is understood at the start.

Ironically, the impact of COVID-19 in 2020 proved advantageous to the quick uptake of Buvidal in some parts of the United Kingdom. It is not uncommon for there to be an extensive time-lag between the licensing of a new medicine, and patients actually receiving it. This is often due to budget restrictions (drug budgets have often already been allocated, and new drugs are expected to be expensive), or the need for local guidelines to be drawn up to ensure the right patients receive the new medication. However, as a result of the extensive and prolonged social distancing restrictions imposed as a result of the pandemic, a more pragmatic solution was sought. The advantages of a weekly or monthly alternative to daily supervision meant that many more patients have already started treatment with Buvidal, as it requires less frequent social contact and therefore protects both staff and patients. Less frequent pharmacy visits will also help to reduce the bill for supervised consumption.

Whilst it is still early days, the response to this new formulation appears to be extremely positive. Anecdotal reports claim Buvidal to be 'game changing'. First-hand accounts from people who had previously battled for years with the revolving door between treatment and chaotic drug use reporting that Buvidal was, for them and their families, 'life changing' through the reduction of anxiety and craving. Either way, the arrival of a new treatment option in this field where few options are available has to be a positive thing for patients.

Potential disadvantages of Buvidal

The negative aspects of the long acting injections so far appear to be relatively limited, with the main one being pain at the site of the injection which, for many, will be a small price to pay in the great scheme of things. There are a number of sites suitable for injection, and these should be rotated to minimise any problems at the injection sites.

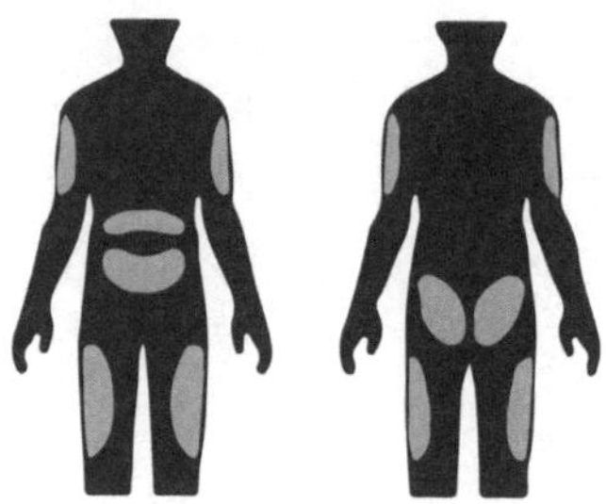

In addition, once the injection had been administered, it cannot be removed. This means that you should weigh up the pros and cons carefully before committing to a treatment which can last for up to a month. Some people are also fearful of needles, and may find having an injection a challenge, even if it is only once a month.

Finally, whilst for many, less contact with healthcare professionals may be seen as a positive step, this may not be the case for everyone. This could result in missing the daily ritual or a loss of daily structure for some people who benefit from both the routine of visiting a pharmacy, and the personal interaction with clinic and pharmacy staff. The therapeutic relationship between healthcare professionals and patients should not be underestimated. That relationship is likely to go beyond the opioid dependence itself. It also provides opportunities for discussing and managing or preventing other physical and psychological conditions. These potential issues are not insurmountable but will need to be considered at the start of treatment, to ensure that sufficient support is in place for the individual who will benefit from it.

Pain Management: As we saw with naltrexone, adequate pain relief with a full opioid agonist may be difficult to achieve in patients receiving buprenorphine. Longer acting formulations, such as Buvidal, may create a greater challenge in such situations. However, experience shows that some pain relief is possible by taking short acting opioids. It is anticipated that the same will be true with Buvidal, but there is currently no data available.

Methadone
Legal Status: Prescription Only Medicine
Class A; Schedule 2 Controlled Drug/Medicine (CD)
Typical maintenance dose: The product licence states 40 – 60mg/ day but the *Orange Guidelines* recommends a maintenance dose of between 60 – 120mg/ day

Brand Name: Methadose®, Metharose®, Physeptone®. Liquids come in several colours: Green (most common), brown or blue. Sugar-free formulations are available

Methadone is a synthetic opioid agonist which is licensed for treating opioid addiction and mild to moderate pain. In the United Kingdom, methadone is available in the following formulations:

- Oral solution usually 1mg/ml (including sugar free). Other higher concentrations are available, but there are obvious risks involved in making errors when switching between strengths and they are not recommended
- Solution for injecting (The use of injectable methadone for this indication must be initiated by physicians with adequate expertise and experience in addiction therapy)
- Tablets (The licence states the tablets are for use for moderate to severe pain only, but they are often used instead of liquids when a person on methadone goes on holiday)

Methadone has been around for well over half a century. To give you a little bit of history, methadone was initially developed as an analgesic in Germany in 1937 to try to combat shortages of morphine and was patented in 1944. It is believed to have been first used as an analgesic in the United Kingdom in 1947, but its effect on respiratory depression made its use problematic. However, it was not used as a treatment for addiction until the 1960s, when two pioneering American psychiatrists, Dr Vincent Dole and Marie Nyswander found that they could stabilise and maintain opiate addicts without having to continually increase the dose.

Since then, methadone has become a well-established treatment throughout the world and there has been an enormous amount of research evidence into its use as both a maintenance and detoxification medication. This has established it as the 'gold-standard' treatment for opioid treatment.

However, despite its status as one of the most researched pharmaceutical treatments in the world, methadone carries with it a lot of negative press. A lot of this may be based around the stereotyping of drug users queuing in some pharmacies every day to receive their supervised dose of 'green liquid', mixed with deep rooted beliefs that 'people who use drugs do not contribute to society and should just be able to stop'. I am hoping that anyone reading this book who harboured these prejudices will now have a better understanding of what brings people to this point in their lives. After all, no one sits down with their careers adviser at school and announces that it is their burning ambition to be dependent upon drugs.

There is also a negative perception about methadone amongst drug users. There are widely held beliefs that 'methadone acts as a chemical cosh that rots your teeth and gets in your bones'. It is also believed to be more addictive than heroin and harder to come off. Methadone is also considered to be extremely dangerous due to headline-grabbing news involving fatal overdoses, especially accidental overdoses of children. I will attempt to unpick these concerns and create some kind of balance, starting with the fact that all medicines will have had to have passed rigorous tests before being allowed on to the market, and methadone is no different. There is an old cliché that says, 'guns don't kill people, people do', and again, methadone is no different. Unfortunately, the very nature of addiction means that the normal rules of engagement around medication compliance are often not followed. However, if used correctly, methadone can be a valuable tool that can reduce criminal behaviour, HIV infection rates, injection-related risk-taking behaviour, illicit opioid use and save lives!

Methadone is a long acting opioid agonist: The fact that it is a full opioid agonist means that when it binds with the opioid receptors, it results in the usual effects of euphoria, lower blood pressure, sedation etc. It can also cause respiratory depression at higher doses and other potentially serious side-effects, such as constipation.

The correct dose of methadone will enable you to start to manage the rest of your life. It can free you up from the daily routine of sourcing, using and recovering from drugs and allow you to start to breathe again and make positive changes. If methadone suits you well, it may reflect the fact that you have other deeper, entrenched challenges in your life that need to be addressed. Being on methadone will *help* you to do that but it will not be a cure – and you don't want to let the tail wag the dog!

You want to use methadone to achieve your personal treatment goals, and if these include abstinence, then to reduce it and ultimately stop. The fact that methadone is long-acting also means that there is an increased risk of death from opioid overdose during induction because there will be a delay in the methadone reaching the optimum effect. The level in the body builds up quite slowly over time, and it takes 3-4 days of daily use to reach a stable level. Increasing the dose of methadone too quickly, or taking other drugs on top before this level has been reached, can result in toxicity which may only become apparent several days later. As the dose has to be increased slowly, it can take up to four weeks (or more) for you to get to be stable on the correct dose, especially if a higher dose is needed. During this period, you may feel uncomfortable and be tempted to 'top up' with other opioids, thereby increasing the risk of overdose further.

Methadone's long duration of action, and in particular its onset of action makes it is less psychologically reinforcing than short acting opioids. If you have been using short-acting opioids regularly and, especially if you have been injecting them, it will take a while to adjust to the different, less intense effect.

People who have a history of injecting often report that they experience a psychological as well as a physical 'high' from injecting. In other words, the actual act of injecting can build up an intense anticipation, which is subsequently rewarded by the drug response itself. Obtaining, preparing and using their injecting paraphernalia (e.g. silver foil, needles, syringes, spoons) can become ritualistic and psychologically addictive. This habit can be extremely difficult to break. Normal, everyday items such as silver foil (used to chase or smoke the heroin), or lemon juice (used to dissolve the heroin prior to 'cooking' to inject it), can trigger this psychological response and lead to an intense craving to use heroin. It can take a while, and plenty of psychological support before this response is extinguished, because it is difficult to adapt the familiar patterns related to needles and self-injection, especially at the start of treatment.

Be mindful also that these triggers can last for many years and can often result in severe cravings or withdrawal symptoms leading to a lapse or full-blown relapse if you are not prepared. Even if you have been abstinent for weeks or months or years, these cravings and withdrawals feel like the real deal. A common example is that strong emotional states such as anger can trigger craving or withdrawal. The craving or withdrawal lasts as long as you are really angry but goes away as you calm down. It may last half an hour, a couple of hours, or even two days in someone who is really angry. Some people relapse when in this state, but the presence of craving or withdrawal symptoms does not mean you need an opioid or that you are undergoing opioid detox again. The craving and withdrawal are automatic responses of the body, that were developed ('conditioned') in the past during the time that you were using opioids. It makes sense that if when you got angry in the past, you would use opioids to cope with your emotional state, and therefore now that you are angry again the body is looking forward to opioids again.

Remember the mountain – that it takes 4-7 years to return to normal after abstinence!

So, let's assume that you have successfully avoided or negotiated the potential pitfalls that can occur at the start of methadone treatment. Once you have achieved your optimum dose, you can remain there for a long time if that is what you need. The *Orange Guidelines* advocate maintenance doses to be in the range of 60mg to 120mg per day, as these doses are generally sufficient to reduce or remove the need for you to use opioids 'on top'. However, if you are less dependent on opioids, lower doses may be appropriate, or consideration can be given to using buprenorphine instead as an alternative OST.

Methadone and Oral Hygiene: Studies have shown that long-term use of opioids leads to an increased desire for sweet-tasting foods. Opioids also restrict the amount of saliva you produce, which exposes your teeth to developing harmful plaque. Furthermore, if you have been experiencing chronic stress, depression or anxiety you may not have been taking the best care of yourself. Methadone is generally prescribed in a liquid formulation and contains various ingredients including sweeteners, thickeners and preservatives, such as glycerol. All opioids taste bitter, and to counteract this some methadone formulations may consist of up to 50% syrup, so it is important to request a sugar-free formulation and perform all the normal routines designed to protect your teeth and gums.

Methadone and overdose

It is extremely easy for an opioid-naïve person to overdose on methadone. As little as 10mg can kill a child, and less than 50mg can kill an adult. Using other drugs that can cause respiratory depression will increase that risk. The supervised consumption of methadone every day is one strategy used to safeguard people from deliberate or accidental overdose. However, for many people who are stable on a regular dose, this can cause unnecessary restrictions to leading a normal life. Remember that if methadone is involved in an overdose situation, you need to call an ambulance and that you may need multiple doses of naloxone, as the rescue- effect of naloxone will wear off faster than the depressant effects of methadone wears off.

Methadone as a detox medication

Methadone detoxification is likely to be a longer process than with buprenorphine, especially if you are being maintained within the recommended dose range of 60-120mg.

The *Orange Guidelines* estimate that you can reduce your methadone down to zero in around 12 weeks based on a reduction rate of around 5mg every one to two weeks, and that many people find it easier to reduce the dose quicker at the start of the process. The fact that methadone is a liquid means that doses can be titrated very accurately, and you can have more flexibility around dosing. The flip side is that it can become all too easy to decrease by such tiny increments that the process appears never-ending, a little like a set of Russian dolls. If do you find yourself starting to struggle with difficult emotions and thoughts, you may be encouraged to stop reducing the dose, or even to increase it slightly, in order to allow you to cope with how you are feeling. Remember, you may start to feel things you have not felt in years, so be kind to yourself. Many people do find that they start to struggle with withdrawal symptoms at some point. If this occurs at or below 60mgs of methadone it may be worth considering switching to buprenorphine for the remainder of your detoxification, as buprenorphine is easier to reduce and is associated with milder withdrawal symptoms.

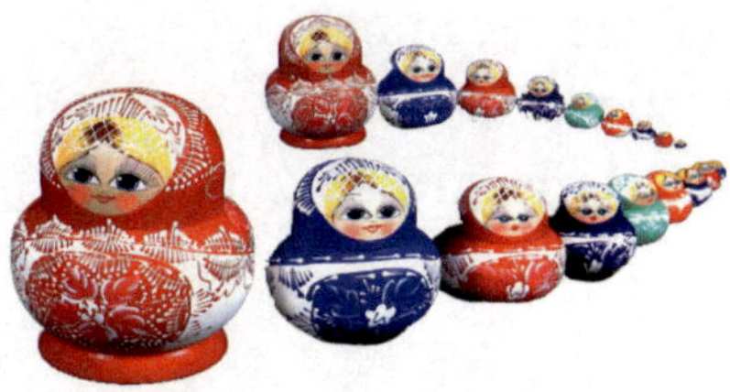

In the previous chapter, I also talked about protracted withdrawal. This can occur at the end of the detox and may last for weeks, months or longer, especially if you have been using high doses of opioids for a long period of time. You may need to continue with symptomatic medicines to help with the longer lasting withdrawal symptoms. It is also worth considering that the opioids you have been taking, maybe at high doses and for a long period of time, may have been masking underlying conditions, including pain e.g. toothache and back pain.

If you continue to feel unwell a few weeks after you have stopped taking opioids it would be worth speaking to your doctor to rule out any other illnesses or injuries, including blood-borne viruses.

Methadone or buprenorphine?

Hopefully you now have a good overview of the pros and cons of the two recommended treatments for both OST and opioid detoxification. Remember, you can play a big part in the decision about which one is most suitable for you, so I have put the key points in the opposite table:

If you wish to find out more about these, or any other medicine, The Electronic Medicines Compendium (EMC) contains up to date, easily accessible information about medicines licensed for use in the UK. EMC website has more than 14,000 documents, all of which have been checked and approved by either the UK or European government agencies which license medicines. You can find the EMC at www.medicines.org.uk.

*** 40% of people experience withdrawal symptoms 24 hours after the last dose of methadone, although most people cope with it. Methadone is therefore not suitable for people who are fast metabolisers, as the effect of the methadone will wear off even quicker.*

	Methadone	Buprenorphine
Severity of dependence	May suit people with longer-term dependence who have more serious underlying psychological issues	May suit people with shorter, less severe dependence who prefer to feel 'more normal'. May not be suitable for people requiring the equivalence of more than 60-80mgs of methadone daily
Starting treatment	Can take 2 to 4 weeks to stabilise onto the appropriate dose	Can be stabilised quicker as the risk of overdose is significantly less. However, there is a risk of precipitated withdrawal if you start taking buprenorphine too soon after your last dose of opioid
Maintenance treatment	Once a day. Initially supervised**	Once a day or at higher doses once every other day.
Overdose risk	High, due to full agonist effect. Risks are higher during the induction period, if you have a reduced or stopped the methadone and also if taken with other opioids or alcohol, benzodiazepines etc	Low, even in people with a low dose of buprenorphine due to the ceiling effect on respiratory depression. However, risks increase if detoxed completely or taken with alcohol, benzodiazepines etc. Buprenorphine also blocks the effect of other opioids
Use in pregnancy	Methadone has been widely used for many years without apparent ill consequence. However, it should only be used during pregnancy if the potential benefit outweighs the potential risk to the unborn baby. Often given twice daily in the third trimester because of more rapid metabolism	Buprenorphine should only be used during pregnancy if the potential benefit outweighs the potential risk to the unborn baby
Minimum age for treatment	18 years or above	16 years or above
Detoxification	Longer detoxification process. May be worth switching to buprenorphine	Shorter, less severe detoxification process
Relapse prevention	You must wait at least 7 to 10 days before starting naltrexone	You should wait 3 to 4 days before starting treatment with naltrexone

CHAPTER 8
The 'Legal Stuff'

As we draw this book to a close, I would like to provide you with some of the more technical and legal information which has been touched upon in some of the chapters, as well as some useful websites which will help you to expand your knowledge or obtain support.

So, to begin with, I have mentioned that treatment may, at some point, involve a number of medicines which may be prescribed either 'off-label' or without a licence; for example, clonidine. It is therefore important that you are aware of the extra checks and balances that are in place to ensure they are prescribed as safely as possible:

- Here in the UK, *the Medicines Act 1968* is the piece of government legislation which controls the use of medicines within the UK and the Medicines and Healthcare products Regulatory Agency (MHRA) is **responsible for monitoring the safety of all medicine**.
- All medicines have side effects and in order for a medicine to be licensed by the MHRA, it must demonstrate that:
    - It is effective in treating the condition for which it is licensed
    - The benefits of using the medicine outweigh the risks
    - It has been manufactured to appropriate quality standards. This is known as Good Manufacturing Practice (GMP)
    - When given to patients, each medicine is accompanied by appropriate information, such as a Patient Information Leaflet (PIL). Packaging is also designed to safeguard against tampering and counterfeiting. This ensures that the patient receives a genuine, quality-assured product
- Patients, the general public and healthcare professionals (such as doctors, nurses and pharmacists) can and should report any serious side-effects to the MHRA, even if these side effects are

already well known. Side effects can be reported online or by post via the MHRA's 'Yellow Card Scheme'. The MHRA will continually review the side effect profile of a medicine and may change or revoke a licence if the 'risk/benefit' balance changes

Use of off-label or unlicensed medications

The General Medical Council (GMC) is the independent regulator for doctors in the UK. The GMC (online) states:

'You are responsible for the prescriptions that you sign. You must only prescribe drugs when you have adequate knowledge of your patient's health. And you must be satisfied that the drugs serve your patient's need.'

The doctor or other prescriber should usually prescribe licensed medicines in accordance with the terms of their licence. However, they may prescribe unlicensed medicines where, on the basis of an assessment of the individual patient, they have concluded for medical reasons, that it is necessary to do so to meet the specific needs of the patient. The doctor or other prescriber must give patients (or their parents or carers) sufficient information about the medicines they propose to prescribe to allow the patient to make an informed decision and must always answer questions from patients (or their parents or carers) about medicines fully and honestly. If the doctor or other prescriber intends to prescribe unlicensed medicines where that is not routine or if there are suitably licensed alternatives available, they should explain this to the patient, and their reasons for doing so.

Some medicines are routinely used outside the terms of their licence, for example clonidine for detoxification. Where prescribing unlicensed medicines is supported by authoritative clinical guidance, the doctor or other prescriber needs to describe in general terms to the patient why the medicine is not licensed for the proposed use or patient population.

Prescribing unlicensed medicines may be necessary where a suitably licensed medicine that would meet the patient's need is not available at all or is not available in the dose or formulation required or is not licensed for that particular age range (e.g. a child). It may also occur when the prescribing forms part of a properly approved research project.

When prescribing an unlicensed medicine the doctor or other prescriber must be satisfied that there is sufficient evidence or experience of using the medicine to demonstrate its safety and efficacy; take responsibility for prescribing the medicine and for overseeing the patient's care, monitoring, and any follow up treatment, or ensure that arrangements are made for another suitable doctor to do so; and make a clear, accurate and legible record of all medicines prescribed and, where they are not following common practice, their reasons for prescribing an unlicensed medicine.

Buyer beware - the risks of counterfeit and online pharmaceuticals

As more people use the internet to understand their health issues, some also go online to buy medication – prescription-only medicines or otherwise. In recent years there has been an explosion of websites offering medicines for sale online. As a result, the supply of counterfeit drugs has become a multi-billion-pound industry. The World Health Organisation (WHO) estimates that possibly 1% of medicines in developed countries are either counterfeit or substandard, rising to 10% in low and middle-income countries and as high as 30% on the African continent.

Seeking information and support online may be especially attractive for people using illicit drugs. Using the internet to help maintain a regular supply may also be attractive to people experiencing opioid addiction, where access to drugs through legitimate channels is, quite rightly, severely restricted. Unfortunately, desperation may lead people to go to extreme measures to try to obtain drugs, including sourcing them via the internet, where there are plenty of unscrupulous individuals waiting to exploit their vulnerabilities to the full. Before you consider sourcing medications in this way, bear in mind that there are strict regulations which pharmaceutical companies, not to mention pharmacies, must comply with before a patient can receive medication. If you still intend sourcing medicines online, here is a check list which the NHS has produced which will help you to avoid some of the pitfalls:

- ✓ Many online pharmacies are unregistered, so buying from them is potentially unsafe. The General Pharmaceutical Council (GPhC) operates an internet pharmacy logo scheme to help you to identify legitimate online pharmacies. In addition, virtual pharmacies should be connected to an actual "bricks and mortar" pharmacy with a real address and contact details, which will help you to verify that they are legitimate
- ✓ Medication from an unregistered website or pharmacy could also be dangerous because it might be out-of-date, substandard, stored incorrectly, or simply fake. Fake medication can cause real harm to your health, as it may not actually contain the active ingredient that you want or, if it does, it may not

be in the correct quantity. All medicines also contain other compounds, such as bulk-forming and coating agents (used to manufacture tablets), preservatives and colourings. All of these ingredients also need to comply with GMP and may also have the potential to cause side effects, such as allergic reactions.

- ✓ Most medications which treat opioid dependence are likely to be prescription-only medicines (POMs). In order to dispense a POM, an online pharmacy must receive a legally valid prescription from your prescriber. This must be either a paper or official electronic prescription. An emailed prescription is not sufficient
- ✓ Your pharmacist and prescriber should be aware of any other medications or health issues you may have before dispensing your medication. This minimises the risk of you developing any potentially serious side-effects caused either by the drug they are dispensing, or as a result of the new drug interacting with any other medication you may be taking (prescribed or otherwise). This extra layer of safety may not be possible via an online service, exposing you to potentially serious consequences

Remember that the policies and procedures mentioned above also apply to non-prescription drugs, including medicines such as paracetamol and ibuprofen, which can be purchased from non-pharmacy retail outlets. Please think carefully before you source any medicine other than from an established, bona fide supplier or prescriber.

Controlled Drugs

The term 'Controlled Drug' is defined by *the Misuse of Drugs Act 1971* ("the Act") as 'any substance or product for the time being specified in Part I, II or III of Schedule 2 of the Misuse of Drugs Act 1971'. Controlled drugs are subject to strict legal controls regarding how they are prescribed, supplied, stored and destroyed and are classified as A, B or C. The *British National Formulary (BNF)* provides the following list:

- **Class A** includes alfentanil, cocaine, diamorphine hydrochloride (heroin), dipipanone hydrochloride, fentanyl, lysergide (LSD), methadone hydrochloride, 3, 4-methylenedioxymethamfetamine (MDMA, 'ecstasy'), morphine, opium, oxycodone hydrochloride, pethidine hydrochloride, phencyclidine, remifentanil, and class B substances when prepared for injection.
- **Class B** includes oral amfetamines, barbiturates, cannabis, *Sativex*®, codeine phosphate, dihydrocodeine tartrate, ethylmorphine, glutethimide, ketamine, nabilone, pentazocine, phenmetrazine, and pholcodine.
- **Class C** includes: certain drugs related to the amfetamines such as benzfetamine and chlorphentermine, buprenorphine, mazindol, meprobamate, pemoline, pipradrol, most benzodiazepines, tramadol hydrochloride, zaleplon, zolpidem tartrate, zopiclone, androgenic and anabolic steroids, clenbuterol, chorionic gonadotrophin (HCG), non-human chorionic gonadotrophin, somatotropin, somatrem, somatropin, gabapentin, and pregabalin.

The *Misuse of Drugs Regulations 2001* (and subsequent amendments), defines the classes of person who are authorised to supply and possess Controlled Drugs while acting in their professional capacities and lays down the conditions under which these activities may be carried out. Drugs are divided into five Schedules, each specifying the requirements governing such activities as import, export, production, supply, possession, prescribing, and record keeping which apply to them.

What are the penalties for possessing or supplying drugs?

The penalties for possession and supply depend on the class the drug belongs to. The maximum penalties under the Misuse of Drugs Act (MDA) are as follows:

Drug class	Possession	Supply
Class A	7 years + fine	Life + fine
Class B	5 years + fine	14 years + fine
Class C	2 years + fine	14 years + fine

Source: DrugWise. Available from www.drugwise.org.uk

The responsibility of the prescriber

The National Institute for Health and Care Excellence (NICE www.bnf.nice.uk) states that the prescriber has three main responsibilities when prescribing drugs likely to cause dependence or misuse:

1. To avoid creating dependence by introducing drugs to patients without sufficient reason

2. To see that the patient does not gradually increase the dose of a drug, given for good medical reasons, to the point where dependence becomes more likely. This tendency is seen especially with hypnotics and anxiolytics. The prescriber should keep a close eye on the amount prescribed to prevent patients from accumulating stocks. A minimal amount should be prescribed in the first instance, or when seeing a patient for the first time

3. To avoid being used as an unwitting source of supply for addicts and being vigilant to methods for obtaining medicines. Methods include visiting more than one doctor, fabricating stories, and forging prescriptions

In addition to the legal restrictions placed upon the supply, administration, storage and dispensing of controlled drugs, further restrictions are in place to ensure that they are used as safely as possible once they have left the pharmacy

Supervised Consumption

Supervised consumption is not a legal requirement under the 2001 Regulations. However, the supervised consumption of a medicine by an appropriate professional is often instigated for both methadone and buprenorphine. I have included this information here in light of the higher risk of overdose with methadone, especially at the start of treatment. For most cases, it will be appropriate for new patients being prescribed methadone or buprenorphine to be required to take their daily doses under the direct supervision of a professional for a period of time. This will allow monitoring of progress and an ongoing risk assessment.

Supervision of the consumption of a Controlled Drug provides the best guarantee that it is being taken as prescribed. It has significantly reduced the amount of methadone-related deaths. It is aimed at keeping you and others safe and should not be viewed as a punishment.

Levels of supervision should be based on an individual risk assessment for, and with, each patient. For many on daily supervised consumption, providing a take-home dose for Sundays is the only practical option, but for others it may be feasible to access a pharmacy that opens seven days a week.

The National Institute for Health and Care Excellence (NICE www.bnf.nice.uk) provides the following information for prescribers of Controlled Drugs:

'Individuals prescribed opioid substitution therapy can take their daily dose under the supervision of a doctor, nurse, or pharmacist during the dose stabilisation phase (usually the first 3 months of treatment), after a relapse or period of instability, or if there is a significant increase in the dose of methadone. Supervised consumption should continue (in accordance with local protocols) until the prescriber is confident that the patient is compliant with their treatment. It is good practice for pharmacists to alert the prescriber when a patient has missed consecutive daily doses.'

Opioids and driving

New drug driving legislation came in to force in England and Wales in 2015 and the Faculty of Pain (www.fpm.ac.uk) have issued the following information :

- It remains illegal in England and Wales to drive when taking prescription medicines, if the medication impairs a patient's ability to drive
- The new offence refers to driving with a specified controlled drug in the body, in excess of a specified limit
- The drugs include licensed medicines, including morphine and methadone, but not other opioids. The specified limits are generally above the normal therapeutic range, so most patients prescribed these drugs are unlikely to be driving with a concentration of a specified drug in their body above the specified limit.
- The new offence has a statutory "medical defence" to protect patients who may test positive for certain specified drugs taken in accordance with the advice of a healthcare professional or the patient information leaflet that accompanies the medicine
- It remains the responsibility of all drivers, including patients, to consider whether they believe their driving may be impaired on every occasion when they drive
- Drivers who tested positive for morphine were between 8 and 32 times more likely to be injured or responsible for a road traffic collision compared with those who did not have a positive test result.

- A patient on high dose morphine (around 200mg/24hours) could be as impaired as someone with blood alcohol around the level above which it is illegal to drive.
- A patient also drinking or taking other sedative drugs could be impaired at a lower morphine dose.
- Patients should be aware that during the period following dose adjustment (up or down) they may be particularly vulnerable to impairment.
- Prescribers of opioid medicines must be aware of the likely impairing effects of the drugs and must advise patients accordingly.
- Although this legislation will particularly impact on patients taking morphine, prescribers should be aware that equi-analgesic doses of other opioids are likely to be equivalently impairing.
- Prescribers should also advise patients of the potentially distracting effects of pain, and other co-morbidities such as fatigue and poor sleep in relation to driving.
- Discussions in relation to drugs and driving must be clearly documented in the medical notes and a copy given to the patient.

RECOMMENDATIONS, RESOURCES AND ADDITIONAL SUPPORT

Recommendations

It is always a difficult thing to make recommendations, but one of the reasons behind writing this book was to provide you with reliable and accurate information. I hope I have done that and have now gained your trust as an author. Whilst the purpose of this book was to explore the background to, and pharmacological treatment options for opioid addiction, trauma is likely to be an integral part of this. As a result, I would like to draw your attention to the following resources:

Trauma Breakthrough

Trauma Breakthrough, which also works under the name Breakthrough is a charity based in Bath and operating across the south-west of England. It provides specialist mental health services and support for adult survivors of abuse and other forms of trauma. It also offers training and consultancy to organisations and individuals who want to learn to support survivors more effectively.
https://www.traumabreakthrough.org

Books

'Breakthrough: The art of surviving' is a book which has been written by Giles Lascelle, Trauma Breakthrough's founder and CEO.
Available from their website or from Amazon.

'The Body Keeps The Score: Mind, Brain and Body in the Transformation of Trauma' by Bessel van der Kolk offers a bold new way of looking at treatment for trauma, moving away from standard talking and drug

therapies and towards an alternative approach that heals mind, brain and body.
Available from Amazon.

Resources

Here is a list of links to website which will direct you to many of the reference documents used throughout the book. Please note, web pages and documents are often moved from the original web address. I have therefore provided the main website e.g. www.gov.uk, as well as the direct link as it was at the time of printing, which will allow you to search for what you are looking for, in the event that it has been moved.

Document/Organisation	Website
British Pain Society	www.britishpainsociety.org/brit-ish-pain-society-publications/pa-tient-publications
Buvidal® (buprenorphine) injection	https://www.buvidal.co.uk
Drug misuse and dependence UK guidelines on clinical management (orange guidelines)	http://www.gov.uk/ https://assets.publishing.service.gov.uk/govern-ment/uploads/system/uploads/attachment_data/file/673978/clini-cal_guidelines_2017.pdf
Electronic Medicines Compendium (EMC)	https://www.medicines.org.uk/emc/
General Medical Council	https://www.gmc-uk.org

Medicines & Healthcare products Regulatory Agency (MHRA)	http://www.gov.uk/ https://www.gov.uk/government/organisations/medicines-and-health-care-products-regulatory-agency
National Institute of Health and Care Excellence	https://www.nice.org.uk
Prenoxad® (naloxone) Injection	http://www.prenoxadinjection.com
Recovery Research Institute	https://www.recoveryanswers.org
Yellow Card Scheme (reporting side effects)	https://yellowcard.mhra.gov.uk/

Additional Support

Organisation That Could Provide Additional Support	
Advocacy After Fatal Domestic Violence	www.aafda.org.uk
Alcohol - AA (Alcoholics Anonymous)	https://www.alcoholics-anonymous.org.uk/Home
Alcohol - Al-Anon	www.al-anonuk.org.uk
Alcohol - Alcohol Concern	www.alcoholconcern.org.uk
Alcohol - Drinkaware	www.drinkaware.co.uk
Adfam (for families)	www.adfam.org.uk

Organisation That Could Provide Additional Support	
Benzodiazepines – BAT (Battle Against Tranquillisers)	www.bataid.org
Benzodiazepines – The Benzo Group Support	www.benzo.org.uk
Child Line	www.childline.org.uk
Citizens Advice Bureau	www.citizensadvice.co.uk
CA (Cocaine Anonymous) UK	www.cauk.org.uk
Disability Rights Commission	https://www.drc.org.uk
Domestic violence - National Centre for Domestic Abuse	www.ncdv.org.uk
Domestic violence - National Domestic Violence Helpline	www.nationaldomesticviolencehelp-line.org.uk
Domestic violence - Men's Advice Line (for domestic violence)	www.mensadviceline.org.uk
Drug Wise	https://www.drugwise.org.uk
FRANK (national drugs helpline)	www.talktofrank.com

Organisation That Could Provide Additional Support	
Help for Heroes (H4H) Hidden Wounds	www.helpforheros.org.uk/hidden-wounds
HIT	www.hit.org.uk
Mental health - MIND	www.mind.org.uk
Mental health - Rethink Mental Illness	www.rethink.org
Mental health - Sane Line	www.sane.org.uk
NA (Narcotics Anonymous)	www.ukna.org
NHS Choices	www.nhs.uk
NSPCC	www.nspcc.org.uk
Relate	www.relate.org.uk
Rape Crisis	www.rapecrisis.org.uk
Refuge	www.refuge.org.uk
Salvation Army	www.salvationarmy.org.uk
Samaritans	www.samaritans.org

Organisation That Could Provide Additional Support	
Shelter National Helpline	www.shelter.org.uk
SMART Recovery UK	www.smartrecovery.org.uk
Smoking - Action on Smoking and Health (ASH)	www.ash.org.uk
Smoking - Smokefree	http://smokefree.nhs.uk

Epilogue
'Beyond the Rainbow'

Writing this book has enabled me to do something I had long considered but never had the confidence to do, and I thank you for indulging my secret desire. If you have drawn just a tiny fraction of the benefit in reading it as I did in writing it, I will be happy. However, now I feel that I must 'come clean', for want of a better expression. If you read my preface, you may recall me making the following statement:

'whilst writing this book will no doubt force me to delve into areas of my life I have attempted to close off, I do not write this as a cathartic 'self-help' manual.'

Well, as I have finally arrived at the finishing line with regards to this venture, I can honestly say that that statement is no longer true. Writing this book coincided unexpectedly with a period of emotional turmoil which, did indeed, send me hurtling towards my own personal Black Hole. As a result, it meant that deadlines were missed, and I battled with the reality that I may not have the focus or the energy to complete this. However, once again thanks to those closest to me, I persevered and am proud to have finally arrived at this point. However, in pressing on, I realised that I was a million miles away from being that 'dispassionate, though empathetic observer' (that may be an oxymoron) I believed I was when faced with the horrors of trauma and addiction in others, in both my personal and professional life. This shocking realisation has led me to finally seek the professional help I had advised many others to seek over the years. Whilst I have not personally been affected by opioid dependence, I have experienced varying degrees of destructive behaviour as a result of my own personal experiences, both as a very young child and as an adult. This has led me to revisit and rewrite certain sections of the book, especially those relating to trauma and stress.

So where am I now? Well, I am writing this from a position of strength and inner calm as I am preparing to see my mother one last time before her funeral next week. Weirdly, I feel my heartbeat increase and my stomach churn as I am typing this, but I am now able to stay focused. I know that my mother is now in a better place. She lived a long, and many would say virtuous life, fulfilling her Catholic duty of having more children than her heart could hold, and sitting in judgement on those around her, especially her 'nearest and dearest'. Her death was as expected, the result of her stubbornly ignoring the advice of family, friends and medical professionals around her, but she died at home, which she would have wanted, and for which I am grateful. She also died the day after Mother's Day and three days after the United Kingdom went in to lock down as a result of the COVID-19 pandemic. The irony of this is that there will be no huge Catholic requiem mass, as there was for my father, who pre-deceased her by seven years. Furthermore, numbers at the graveside burial service will be strictly limited to 'close family' only, and social distancing must be observed at all times – which is a huge relief for me on many levels.

To the outsider, these sentiments may wreak of bitterness, and some, especially those that know me, may be shocked by my words. All I know is that these are my heart-felt thoughts based on a lifetime of sensing and observing. A child always senses when a parent doesn't like them, and I have lived with that feeling, and the absolute belief that nothing I did would ever be good enough, all of my life. This has been compounded by the fact that I have observed others around me who have not behaved well and have, to all intents and purposes, been rewarded for it. I acknowledge that the injustice of this does, indeed, instill a sense of bitterness. However, that is far outweighed by the freedom I now have to continue my journey setting right the self-doubt and low self-esteem that has dogged me all my life. This was something I was unable to do effectively while my mother was alive, as 'dragging up the past' in such an explosive way would, I am certain, have shortened her life. I have been far kinder to her than she has been to me, and I see that as a very positive thing. I am under no illusion that the next stage of my journey will be long and difficult, but I am reliably informed that repairing deep-rooted psychological damage is absolutely possible! I believe that, with lots of support from those closest to me, I will finally be able to move on from the past and learn to live *in* the present and *for* the future.

Acknowledgements

Dr Fergus Law MBChB, BSc and FRCPsych

Before I sign off for the last time, I would like to say a special word of thanks to Dr Fergus Law. Fergus is a highly respected Consultant in Substance Misuse Psychiatry who has also been elected a Fellow of Royal College of Psychiatrists for his contribution to psychiatry. He has sat on several national expert groups and is a regular speaker at national conferences and training events. Fergus has also published 15 peer reviewed original research papers and has also been a peer reviewer and associate editor for several academic journals. He has a particular interest in helping people detoxify and remain abstinent and has written the Samurai Approach to Detoxification from Opiates. He is Medical Director of The Lion Clinic based in the South West of England.

I have been honoured to have known Fergus ever since our paths crossed in Bristol in the early 1990s. Our careers ran in parallel for over 25 years (albeit mine was working for the 'dark side' in the pharmaceutical industry), but I have, for many years, been able to count him as a trusted friend. In addition to providing me with some of the content for this book AND doing me the huge honour of 'sense checking' it prior to publication, Fergus also stepped forward and encouraged me to pursue the path to recovery I am now on. I will be forever grateful to him for this.

Dr Jan Melichar BSc, MB BS, MD, FRCPsych

Jan has had a portfolio career focused around substance misuse and mental health spanning nearly 3 decades. He has had varied roles including academic, private and public health sector and consultancy work. In addition to casting another specialist 'pair of eyes' over the content of this book, he has been able to provide invaluable information based upon his clinical experience using the newer buprenorphine-based treatment options. I have known Jan almost as long as I have known Fergus and will always be grateful for the support he has given me throughout those years.

Dr Joy Bampton BSc (Hons); PhD

Joy holds an Advanced Diploma in Therapeutic Counselling, is an accredited member of BACP and an accredited EMDR practitioner.

Having decided that 2020 was the year for change, I carried out extensive research and decided that the best way forward was to engage in Eye Movement Desensitisation and Re-processing (EMDR). I engaged Joy as my EMDR therapist and began the preparation a few weeks before my mother passed away. This process has been an extremely grueling, terrifying yet fascinating and rewarding experience. No matter how ready I thought I was, nothing could have prepared me for what happened in some of those sessions. Joy has seen me at my worst and most vulnerable state on several occasions, but has kept me safe whilst remaining empathetic, professional and deeply caring throughout. For that I am deeply grateful. We still have a long journey ahead together, but I am more confident knowing she is there with me.

Ethypharm

Ethypharm is a global company and a major player in the field of Drug Delivery Systems. Its UK-based division specialises in the field of opioid addiction, emergency care and sterile injectables. I am extremely grateful to them for allowing me access to their educational resources and for permitting me to include some of their images used to support the safe use of their naloxone formulation Prenoxad®, and their buprenorphine 'wafer', Espranor®. Please note that the 'overdose man' diagram was not designed by Ethypharm.